The Ultimate Recipe for Fitness

SHEILA CLUFF & ELEANOR BROWN

Spa Cuisine
from
The Oaks at Ojai
&
The Palms at Palm Springs

Fitness Publications
Ojai, California

This book is dedicated to all who are searching for their

ULTIMATE RECIPE FOR FITNESS

Copyright ©1990
Second Printing
Revised Edition ©1993 by Sheila Cluff and Eleanor Brown

PUBLISHERS CATALOGING IN PUBLICATION DATA
Cluff, Sheila & Brown, Eleanor

THE ULTIMATE RECIPE FOR FITNESS
Spa Cuisine from The Oaks at Ojai and The Palms at Palm Springs

Includes Index

1, Cooking. 2, Fitness.

ISBN: 0-9618805-4-6

Library of Congress Catalog Card Number: 90-082040

PUBLISHED by: FP   FITNESS PUBLICATIONS
                         1991 Country Place, Ojai, CA 93023

COVER DESIGN AND ART by Itoko Maeno
BOOK DESIGN by Christine Nolt

Printed in the United States of America

FOREWORD

Clearly, health, fitness and well being will dominate the lifestyles of the 90s. The 'Pepsi Generation' has become the 'Fitness Generation'. Nutritious, low fat, calorically controlled eating is now a necessity and will continue to be so. It has been demonstrated that regular aerobic exercise reduces the risk of heart disease, stroke and cancer, more importantly though aerobic exercise greatly improves the quality of life.

It is not difficult to understand that healthy eating and proper exercise improve the quality of our lives. However, it is often difficult to put these concepts into action. Here, at last, is a book that makes health and fitness fun; it contains truly delicious, healthy, down home style, energy boosting recipes. The authors have created good to eat, easy to prepare foods that are good for you. The health principles behind the recipes and the fitness tips are scientifically accurate. The recipes and the fitness tips are entertaining reading. Every time the recipes are used the fitness tips will remind one that exercise is essential, also.

This is a no nonsense approach to health and fitness. There are no gimmicks or unrealistic promises or magic, quick-fix-it claims. This cookbook is definitely for the health conscious, the athlete and the waist watcher. These low fat, low cholesterol, high complex carbohydrate recipes can definitely assist in achieving a nutritionally well balanced diet. The recurring theme here is never say diet, don't feel deprived. These nourishing, great tasting foods will delight the whole family from preschooler to grandpa.

This book is recommended to all who believe that health, vigor and a productive, happy life are essential. It will be a handy reference for students in culinary classes. At Cornell Hotel School, we offer a course entitled 'Contemporary Health Cuisine'; this text will be an invaluable aid for our students.

Read and eat in good health.

Mary H. Tabacchi, Ph.D., R.D.
Professor of Nutrition
School of Hotel Administration
Cornell University

INTRODUCTION

After a Spa vacation at The Oaks at Ojai or The Palms at Palm Springs, guests invariably leave feeling terrific. We have written THE ULTIMATE RECIPE FOR FITNESS, not as a substitute for a spa vacation, but as a way that you can create the spa experience at home.

As many of you know, we have published several books on fitness and nutrition. With each book, we have added topics and information that readers and spa guests have requested. In THE ULTIMATE RECIPE FOR FITNESS, you will find a Twenty Eight Day Dinner Menu and a multitude of valuable fitness tips.

All of the recipes in this book are new or revised and because we know that you are knowledgeable and care about these things, each recipe also includes a breakdown of grams and percentages of fat, protein and carbohydrates, as well as milligrams of sodium.

As you use this book, you will find favorite recipes that will become part of your slim, fit lifestyle. You will also find fitness tips for incorporating exercise into that lifestyle. Be patient with yourself and make these changes slowly, working always for permanent new health habits rather than crash programs. The result should be a permanently slimmer trimmer you.

It is our sincere hope that you find your own 'Ultimate Recipe for Fitness' within the pages of this book.

Sheila and Eleanor

Handwritten notes (top of page):

✓ cookies p. 176 ✓ apple stuff p. 8 & 9 ✓ carrot cake - p 159

receipe notes
tuna salad - p. 79
french cream p 15
salsa - p. 31
potassium broth - p. 66
turkey - p. 133
loaf

CONTENTS

RECIPE INFORMATION AND COOKING TIPS

The following is a list of information that we hope will make it easier for you to understand and find ingredients for these recipes:

APPLE JUICE CONCENTRATE is frozen apple juice with no added water. We use it as a sweetener.

CALORIES listed for each recipe have been rounded to the nearest 0 or 5.

NUTRITIONAL VALUES given at the end of each recipe have the fractions rounded to the nearest whole number. Less than 1/2 gram is shown as a TRACE.

MICROWAVE TEMPERATURES are HIGH unless noted.

LIFETIME CHEESE is the lowfat cheese we use. If you are unable to find it in your area, you will find an order blank in the back of this book. Nonfat cheese may be substituted.

BERNARD JENSEN'S BROTH POWDER is the seasoning we use instead of salt. It is for sale in most health food stores. If you are unable to locate it, there is an order blank in the back of this book.

HAIN STONEGROUND MUSTARD is another salt free seasoning that we would hate to be without. That product is available in most markets.

GARLIC that is microwaved until it pops (about 30 seconds) almost peels itself.

A LEMON that is microwaved for 15 seconds will produce juice more easily.

1% COTTAGE CHEESE is called for in these recipes and the nutrients are figured accordingly. The use of Nonfat Cottage Cheese will further reduce fat and calories.

CANOLA OIL is recommended because it has the least amount of saturated fat (which has been shown to increase cholesterol levels.)

OLIVE OIL has a little more saturated fat than Canola Oil, but we use it in small amounts for flavor. All fats are equally fattening. Use them sparingly.

PEANUT BUTTER is ground peanuts with nothing added. Avoid hydrogenated peanut butter. Hydrogenating fat makes it more saturated.

ZEST is the lightly grated colored part of citrus peel.

DELICIOUS DRESSINGS, DIPS AND SPREADS

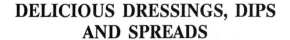

Traditional DRESSINGS, DIPS AND SPREADS tend to rely on fat, salt and sugar for flavor. Since spa cuisine must be low in those unhealthy ingredients, these recipes are invaluable.

They will save you calories daily. As you find your favorites, make them in quantity and keep them available in your freezer. As an example of the importance of this: my husbands favorite dressing is RASPBERRY VINAIGRETTE. As long as I have it in the refrigerator, he uses it on his salads. If I run out and fail to replace it immediately, he slathers undue amounts of mayonnaise on his salads. Since even lowcal mayo has some fat and RASPBERRY VINAIGRETTE has none, the value of keeping the nonfat dressing that he likes in the refrigerator becomes obvious.

Included in this section are jams and marmalades to satisfy your sweet tooth. Use them on toast and crackers instead of butter.

You will find a variety of dressings to help you create wonderful salads. There are great dips to serve with nonfat chips, crackers and crunchy vegetables. Your guests will love you for serving delicious food that won't make them feel fat and heavy.

The sauces and glazes will make your food look beautiful and add so much flavor that you won't miss salt. You will find additional sauces throughout the book, so make up a lot of your favorites and use those to decalorize some of your old recipes as part of your ULTIMATE RECIPE FOR FITNESS.

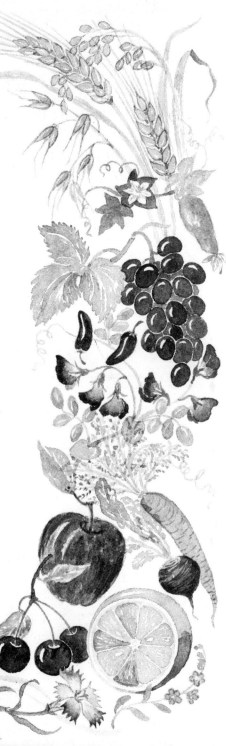

APPLE BUTTER

MAKES 32 ONE TABLESPOON SERVINGS   **15 CALORIES PER SERVING**

2   PIPPIN APPLES
            1. Wash, cut and process in food processor to grate fine.

1/2 C.   APPLE JUICE
1 1/2 TSP. CINNAMON
            2. Combine with apples in sauce pan and cook over low heat until mixture is thick and brown. Stir often.
            3. Place APPLE BUTTER in jam pot and taste.

1/2   LEMON, JUICED
            4. Add to APPLE BUTTER if more tartness is desired.

NOTE: This sugar free jam is a great topping for toast or muffins. Try it on the TRIPLE APPLE OAT BRAN MUFFIN, rice cakes or nonfat yogurt.

SHEILA'S FITNESS TIP: Eat breakfast everyday? People who eat breakfast tend to live longer than those who ignore early morning nourishment. If time is short, eat a TRIPLE APPLE OAT BRAN MUFFIN on the way to work.

CARB 4 GM (94%)   PROTEIN TRACE (1%)   FAT TRACE (4%)   SODIUM TRACE

APPLE CHUTNEY

MAKES 32 ONE TABLESPOON SERVINGS   **15 CALORIES PER SERVING**

2	C.	APPLE, 1/4 INCH DICED	1/2	TSP.	GARLIC, MINCED
1/4	C.	DATES, CHOPPED	1/2	TSP.	FRESH GINGER, MINCED
1/4	C.	RAISINS	1/4	C.	APPLE CIDER VINEGAR
1/4	TSP.	CORIANDER	1/4	C.	APPLE JUICE CONCENTRATE
1/4	TSP.	CUMIN	1/4	C.	WATER

1. Combine in a sauce pan and stir over low heat until liquid is absorbed and apples are tender.

TO MICROWAVE: Combine all ingredients in a 2 quart glass bowl, HALVING THE LIQUID. Microwave for 5 minutes; stir and cook for another 5 minutes. Then stir and check for texture.

2. Cover Chutney and chill.

3. Serve with Indian food and/or rice.

NOTE: This is an extremely simple chutney. You may find that you enjoy the flavors so much that you will use it as a flavor enhancer for many foods. Try it with poultry instead of cranberry sauce. DELICIOUS!

SHEILA'S FITNESS TIP: According to a recent study conducted by THE INSTITUTE FOR AEROBICS RESEARCH, you do not need to be a Marathon Runner to get substantial health benefits from regular exercise. GET OFF YOUR DUFF AND LIVE LONGER is the message in a study quoted in the JOURNAL OF THE AMERICAN MEDICAL ASSOCIATION. Death rates for the least-fit men, 3.4 times higher; women, 4.6 times higher.

CARB 4 GM (96%)   PROTEIN TRACE (2%)   FAT TRACE (1%)   SODIUM TRACE

AVOCADO SALAD DRESSING

MAKES 24 ONE OUNCE SERVINGS   **20 CALORIES PER SERVING**

1/2	C.	AVOCADO, DICED	3		GARLIC CLOVES
1/3	C.	PARMESAN CHEESE, GRATED	2	TSP.	OREGANO
2 1/2	C.	TOMATO JUICE, UNSALTED	2	TSP.	BASIL
3/4	C.	RED WINE VINEGAR			

1. Combine in blender and process until smooth.
2. Place in a jar and refrigerate. (Will keep for a week.)

NOTE: This was developed for the CALORIE CONSCIOUS COBB SALAD found in the SALAD section of this book. However, it is wonderful on any green salad. Oaks Executive Chef David Del Nagro developed an even lighter Avocado Dressing which is also very good. To try it, combine the following:

1	C.	AVOCADO, DICED	1	TSP.	GARLIC
2	C.	ICEBERG LETTUCE, PACKED	3	T.	APPLE CIDER VINEGAR
1/4	C.	SCALLIONS, CHOPPED	2	T.	LEMON JUICE
1/4	C.	PARSLEY, CHOPPED	1	C.	COLD WATER

NOTE: This is best used the day it is made.

SHEILA'S FITNESS TIP: To avoid having a silhouette like an avocado, keep your abdominals strong with CURL UPS: Lie on your back, bend your knees and bring your heels about 12 inches from your buttocks. Place your chin on your chest and hands at the beginning of your thighs. Inhale and as you exhale, lift your torso with your abdominals, sliding your hands up your thighs. Start with 5 and work up to as many as 20.

CARB 3 GM (46%)   PROTEIN 1 GM (11%)   FAT 1 GM (42%)   SODIUM 140 MG

BEAN DIP

25 CALORIES PER SERVING

1/2	C.	ONION	1	TSP.	CUMIN
1	TSP.	GARLIC	1/4	TSP.	OREGANO
1/2	C.	BELL PEPPER	1	TSP.	CHILI POWDER
1/2	C.	TOMATO SAUCE	2	T.	RED WINE
1	C.	KIDNEY BEANS, COOKED	4	OZ.	TOFU
		(IF CANNED, RINSE)			

1. Combine all ingredients in food processor and puree.
2. Place in sauce pan, bring to simmer and cook and stir for 5 minutes.
TO MICROWAVE: Place ingredients in glass bowl or cup and microwave
2-3 minutes.
3. Serve as a dip with tortilla chips or as a filling for a burrito.

NOTE: This is a great change from cheese based dips and when we serve it, we get raves. Try topping it with a bit of lowcal sour cream and be sure to make your own tortilla chips. (Cut corn tortillas and crisp them on a cookie sheet in a 350 oven.)

SHEILA'S FITNESS TIP: Use ENVIRONMENTAL CONTROL in your office. Stock your office refrigerator with low-calorie high fiber snacks like our BEAN DIP. You'll be eating healthier and might even lose some excess body weight since you won't be as tempted by the fatty, sugary snacks in the vending machine down the hall.

CARB 4 GM (58%)   PROTEIN 2 GM (27%)   FAT TRACE (15%)   SODIUM 3 MG

BUTTERMILK HERB DRESSING

MAKES 12 ONE OUNCE SERVINGS   **15 CALORIES PER SERVING**

1 1/4	C.	BUTTERMILK
6	T.	CUCUMBER, SEEDED AND GRATED
3	T.	SCALLIONS, MINCED
1	T.	PARSLEY, MINCED
1	T.	HAIN STONE GROUND MUSTARD
2	TSP.	LEMON JUICE
1/4	TSP.	PEPPER, GROUND
1/4	TSP.	DILLWEED

1. Combine all ingredients and MIX BY HAND.
2. Chill overnight and serve on fresh greens.

NOTE: Be sure to resist the temptation to put the whole thing in your blender lest it turn an unattractive color. This really does need to be hand mixed.

SHEILA'S FITNESS TIP: THE BEST PLACE TO WALK: City, country, mountains and the beach all present unique opportunities for THE FITNESS WALKER. But the best place? Your own neighborhood because it's convenient and just a few steps away.

CARB 1 GM (52%)   PROTEIN 1 GM (30%)   FAT TRACE (18%)   SODIUM 44 MG

CRAB DIP

MAKES 32 ONE TABLESPOON SERVING   20 CALORIES PER SERVING

2 OZ.   **SHARP CHEDDAR CHEESE, (ROOM TEMPERATURE WORKS BEST)**
1. Place in food processor and process to small crumbs.

1 1/2 C.   **LOWFAT COTTAGE CHEESE (1%)**
2. Add to food processor and process smooth.

1/2 C.   **IMITATION CRAB MEAT, RINSED OR FRESH CRAB MEAT**
2 T.   **SCALLIONS, CUT**
2 T.   **FRESH PARSLEY**
1 T.   **PARMESAN CHEESE**
3. Add to food processor and process to mix. Use a pulse technique to retain the texture of the last ingredients.
4. Place in a bowl, cover and refrigerate.
5. Use as a dip with your favorite whole grain crackers, celery or artichoke leaves.

NOTE: This can be formed in balls, garnished with shredded crab and/or parsley and served on a ring of parsley. It is a sure fire success on an hors d'oeuvre table. If there should be any leftover, fold in some whipped egg white and bake it as a Crab Souffle...Delicious!

SHEILA'S FITNESS TIP: A regular exercise program takes your thoughts away from run of the mill worries and makes you feel mellow...PLUS it keeps you in great shape! Vary your program and try new activities before the old ones become dull.

CARB TRACE (10%)   **PROTEIN 26 GM (56%)**   **FAT 1 GM (34%)**   **SODIUM 67 MG**

CREAMY CHEESE

1 OZ.   **MOZZARELLA CHEESE (PART SKIM MILK)**
1. Place in food processor and process to crumble fine.

1 1/2 C.   **LOWFAT COTTAGE CHEESE (1%)**
2. Add to food processor and process as smooth as cream cheese.
3. Place in a covered dish and store in refrigerator.
4. Use as a spread on crackers, fruit or vegetables.

OPTIONAL ADDITIONS:
1/4 C.   **SCALLIONS, CHOPPED FINE**
2 T.   **FRESH MINCED DILL WEED**
1 T.   **PARMESAN CHEESE, GRATED**
1 TSP. **HAIN STONE GROUND MUSTARD**

NOTE: This is my all time favorite calorie and fat saver. Use any cheese you like in place of the Mozzarella, remembering that if you use a higher fat cheese, the calories and fat percentage will be higher. For example, if you use cream cheese, your fat percentage will go up to 56% and the calories will increase to 23 per tablespoon. Try some of this spread on whole grain crackers along with fresh fruit for a quick and delicious lunch.

> SHEILA'S FITNESS TIP: Stretch after a mild warm up but stretch slowly, never bobbing or bouncing. Stretch, hold and then stretch just a little bit more. Make stretching a part of YOUR ULTIMATE RECIPE FOR FITNESS.

CARB TRACE (10%)   PROTEIN 26 GM (56%)   FAT 1 GM (34%)   SODIUM 67 MG

FRENCH CREAM

MAKES 24 ONE OUNCE SERVINGS   **10 CALORIES PER SERVING**

3	C.	LOWFAT COTTAGE CHEESE (1%)
1/4	C.	YOGURT, NONFAT

1. Combine in blender or food processor and process until mixture is smooth and creamy.

2. Place in a bowl or small covered dish and leave at room temperature for 6 hours. Drain off any water that appears.

3. Place in refrigerator for at least 10 hours.

4. Use as topping for desserts, vegetables, potatoes, pasta or rice. Sweeten or add herbs as desired.

NOTE: This deliciously creamy mixture becomes more mellow as it ages, however it may be used right after it is mixed. It will keep for three weeks in your refrigerator.

SHEILA'S FITNESS TIP: Exercise raises self esteem. Accomplishing a challenging workout increases optimism. Why? Because exercise induced endorphins stimulate a sense of well-being and may promote anti-fatigue feelings.

CARB 1 GM (18%)   **PROTEIN 4 GM (69%)**   **FAT TRACE (13%)**   **SODIUM 111 MG**

ITALIAN DRESSING

3		GARLIC CLOVES
2	TSP.	OREGANO
2	TSP.	BASIL

1. With food processor running, drop in garlic and herbs to mince and mix.

1/3	C.	OLIVE OIL
1/3	C.	PARMESAN CHEESE
2 1/2	C.	TOMATO JUICE
1/2	C.	RED WINE VINEGAR

2. Add to food processor and process to mix well.

3. Store dressing in a covered container and use on salads or as a marinade for vegetables.

NOTE: This is an excellent dressing for a Pasta Salad and has been a favorite at The Oaks and The Palms for years. Some fresh Basil and/or Oregano makes a attractive garnish and enhances flavor.

SHEILA'S FITNESS TIP: Avoid crash diets; they don't work. There may be immediate weight loss, but most likely it's water weight. Use the recipes in this book and increase your intake of crunchy salads with dressings like this one.

CARB 1 GM (23%)   PROTEIN TRACE (7%)   FAT 1 GM (70%)   SODIUM 10 MG

LITE ORIENTAL SAUCE

MAKES 16 ONE TABLESPOON SERVINGS   **5 CALORIES PER SERVING**

3/4	C.	WATER
1	T.	ARROWROOT
2	T.	SOY SAUCE, LOW SODIUM
1	T.	BLACK STRAP MOLASSES

1. Combine in a small sauce pan and cook and stir over low heat until sauce is clear and thickened.

TO MICROWAVE: Combine ingredients in a 2 cup glass measuring cup and microwave for 2 minutes.

NOTE: This simple recipe is a blessing for those who must restrict their sodium and love to pour on the Soy Sauce. It keeps well in the refrigerator in a covered cruet. Use as desired as a substitute for high sodium soy sauce.

SHEILA'S FITNESS TIP: A man should not be more than 19 to 21 percent body fat and a woman no more than 20 to 22 percent body fat. These are general measurements. However, if you are considerably over the percentages above, you may be at risk regardless of the numbers on your bathroom scale.

CARB 1 MG (100%)   PROTEIN 0 MG   FAT 0 MG   SODIUM 1 MG

MAYONNAISE & VARIATIONS

MAKES 28 ONE TABLESPOON SERVINGS   **15 CALORIES PER SERVING**

1		EGG
1 1/3	C.	LOWFAT COTTAGE CHEESE (1%)
2	TSP.	RED WINE VINEGAR

1. Combine in blender and process smooth.

1	T.	CANOLA OIL

2. Add slowly to blender contents with blender running.
3. Store in covered container in refrigerator.

NOTE: Variations are easily made by adding one or two ingredients to the basic recipe. To produce a marvelous SAUCE FOR COOKED VEGETABLES, add fresh lemon juice or Balsamic Vinegar to taste. The more lemon juice or vinegar you add, the lower will be the fat content and calories. If you haven't made your own mayonnaise, you can buy one of the low calorie commercial brands and proceed as above. For a great GUACAMOLE, add 1/4 cup mashed avocado and 1/2 cup fresh chopped tomato to 1/4 cup of this mayonnaise. If you like more heat, substitute tomato salsa for the fresh tomato.

SHEILA'S FITNESS TIP: Don't 'give up' all your favorite foods—instead look for a lighter substitute or simply eat less of some of your old favorites.

CARB 1 GM (17%)   PROTEIN 2 GM (57%)   FAT TRACE (26%)   SODIUM 55 MG

MEXICAN SALAD DRESSING

MAKES 16 ONE OUNCE SERVINGS   **10 CALORIES PER SERVING**

1	C.	WHITE VINEGAR
1	TSP.	HONEY
1	T.	LEMON JUICE
1 3/4	C.	WATER
1	T.	CANOLA OIL
1/4	TSP.	BLACK PEPPER, GROUND

1. Combine in a sauce pan and heat.

1	T.	ARROWROOT
1/4	C.	ORANGE JUICE

2. Whisk together and then into sauce pan.
3. Cook and stir to thicken mixture.
4. Chill and serve on greens with fruit.
TO MICROWAVE: Mix all ingredients in a 4 cup glass cup and microwave
2 minutes. Whisk. If mixture is not yet thick microwave for another half minute.

NOTE: This has been a favorite dressing at The Oaks for years but this is the first time the recipe has been in a book. See the recipe for ORANGE ONION SALAD in the SALAD SECTION of this book.

SHEILA'S FITNESS TIP: A sound, balanced, nutritional program that cuts out unnecessary sugars and fats is far more effective than popping vitamin pills.

CARB 2 GM (51%)   PROTEIN TRACE (3%)   FAT 1 GM(45%)   SODIUM 2 MG

NONFAT YOGURT CREAM CHEESE

MAKES 12 ONE TABLESPOON SERVINGS   **10 CALORIES PER SERVING**

1 C. **NONFAT YOGURT**
1. Place in a large strainer or cheese cloth lined colander.
2. Arrange strainer or colander over a larger container so that the bottom of the strainer or colander is an inch or two above the bottom of the container.
3. Set the container in your refrigerator for three hours or overnight.
4. Place the resulting cream cheese in a crock or covered container and use as you would regular cream cheese.

NOTE: Try adding herbs to this for use as a dip or spread. It is absolutely delicious topped with Orange Marmalade or any of the fruit jams or preserves in this section. It is hard to imagine anything better for afternoon tea than an Orange Oat Muffin halved and spread with this cheese and topped with a bit of Orange Marmalade. Many people assure me that they prefer this to regular cream cheese.

SHEILA'S FITNESS TIP: Before moving a muscle—after the alarm rings—start the day with a GIANT stretch. Exaggerate every area of your anatomy. Stretch for one minute.

CARB 1 GM (56%)   PROTEIN 1 GM (42%)   FAT TRACE (2%)   SODIUM 10 MG

OAKS TOMATO SALSA

MAKES 64 ONE TABLESPOON SERVINGS   **10 CALORIES PER SERVING**

1	C.	ONION, CHOPPED
1	TSP.	GARLIC, MINCED
1/2	TSP.	OLIVE OIL

1. Combine in a skillet and saute until onion is clear.

1/2	TSP.	OREGANO	1/4	TSP.	GROUND SAGE
1/2	TSP.	CUMIN	1/2	TSP.	DRY MUSTARD

2. Sprinkle over onion and continue cooking

1	C.	TOMATILLOS, CHOPPED	1/4	C.	JALAPENOS, MINCED

3. Add to skillet and continue cooking until tomatillos are tender.

3	LB.	TOMATOES, CHOPPED	4	OZ.	TOMATO PUREE
6	OZ.	CANNED GREEN CHILIES, CHOPPED	2	T.	CIDER VINEGAR
2	T.	CILANTRO, MINCED (OPTIONAL)	1	T.	LEMON JUICE
2	T.	SCALLIONS, MINCED	2	T.	PARSLEY, MINCED

4. Mix all ingredients in a large bowl and store in a one quart jar. Put the surplus in a covered dish and use as a very flavorful sauce on almost anything.

NOTE: This is Oaks Executive Chef, David Del Nagros recipe. Our Oaks guests are pleased to find that they can have this as a seasoning any time they want and as much as they want. If you find this too hot for your taste, try our milder SIMPLE SALSA in RECIPES FOR FITNESS FOR VERY BUSY PEOPLE.

SHEILA'S FITNESS TIP: When you wake up, sit on the edge of your bed, bring your shoulders up to your ears (or as high as possible), then drop them to loosen your upper back. Repeat five times.

CARB 1 GM (74%)   PROTEIN TRACE (14%)   FAT TRACE (12%)   SODIUM 2 MG

PINEAPPLE MARMALADE

MAKES 16 ONE TABLESPOON SERVINGS   10 CALORIES PER SERVING

1   **ORANGE (LARGE NAVEL PREFERRED)**
1. Wash, cut and place in food processor.
2. Process to chop coarsely.

1/4 C.   **APPLE JUICE CONCENTRATE**
1/4 C.   **RAISINS**
3. Combine with orange in a sauce pan and cook until the orange peel is cooked. Taste a piece.

1 C.   **PINEAPPLE, CANNED UNSWEETENED OR FRESH**
4. Cut into 1/4 inch pieces and add to pan for the last 5 minutes of cooking.
5. Cool and use on muffins or toast.

NOTE: This would also be delicious with Indian food or as a condiment with your Easter Ham. Cover it well and store in your refrigerator. For ORANGE MARMALADE, eliminate the pineapple and use dates instead of raisins.

SHEILA'S FITNESS TIP: Keep your posture tall and straight, abdominals tucked in, and wrap a towel around the sole of your right foot. Hold the ends of the towel in your hands. Place your left leg in a comfortable position. Now, extend your right leg, keeping a slight flex to the knee, and feel the stretch in your hamstring. Hold for a count of 15, release, and switch legs.

CARB 3 GM (95%)   PROTEIN TRACE (3%)   FAT TRACE (2%)   SODIUM 1 MG

PINEAPPLE SALSA

MAKES 12 ONE OUNCE SERVINGS   **15 CALORIES PER SERVING**

1/2	LB.	TOMATILLOS
2	T.	SCALLIONS, CUT
1/2	TSP.	CORIANDER
1/4	TSP.	GARLIC POWDER
1/2	T.	RICE VINEGAR

1. Combine in a food processor and chop to a relish consistency using on/off technique. Take care not to over process into mush.

1	C.	PINEAPPLE, COARSELY CHOPPED
1/2	C.	GREEN CHILIES, CHOPPED
1	T.	BERNARD JENSEN'S BROTH POWDER

2. Combine in a sauce pan with food processor contents and bring to a simmer.

3. Remove from heat and chill 2-3 hours or overnight.

4. Serve with fish or poultry.

NOTE: I developed this recipe to go with the COLD POACHED SALMON recipe in this book. When the SOUTHERN CALIFORNIA CULINARY GUILD had lunch at The Oaks, it was the most requested recipe.

SHEILA'S FITNESS TIP: To tone the buttocks, the next time you climb a flight of stairs, pretend you are holding a gold coin between the cheeks of your seat. Don't drop it until you reach the top.

CARB 2 GM (78%)   PROTEIN TRACE (19%)   FAT TRACE (3%)   SODIUM TRACE

PINEAPPLE SWEET & SOUR SAUCE

MAKES 20 ONE OUNCE SERVINGS   35 CALORIES PER SERVING

| 10 | OZ. | CAN OF UNSWEETENED PINEAPPLE CHUNKS |

1. Drain juice into a sauce pan, reserving pineapple.

2	T.	WATER
2	T.	HONEY
3	T.	SOY SAUCE, LOW SODIUM

2. Add and cook and stir over low heat to thicken sauce.

TO MICROWAVE: Using a 4 cup glass measuring cup or bowl, place above ingredients in microwave for 3 minutes on high. Remove and stir well with a wire whisk or fork. If sauce is not yet clear and thick, microwave for another minute.

1/2	C.	BELL PEPPER, SLICED THIN
1/2	C.	ONION, HALVED AND SLICE THIN OR COARSELY CHOPPED.
1	C.	FIRM FRESH TOMATO, HALVED AND SLICED
		THE RESERVED PINEAPPLE

3. Add to sauce and serve or cook for 1 to 2 minutes and serve.

NOTE: This may be chilled and served as a salad dressing with seafood or poultry. It is delicious served hot over brown rice, topped with a few toasted cashews, almonds or walnuts. Add some shrimp for a marvelous SWEET AND SOUR SHRIMP.

SHEILA'S FITNESS TIP: Being fit will help you handle the stressors in your life. As your fitness level improves you will feel more in control and that will enable you to glide right over stressful situations.

CARB 8 GM (88%)   PROTEIN TRACE (8%)   FAT TRACE (4%)   SODIUM 3 MG

RASPBERRY VINAIGRETTE

MAKES 12 ONE OUNCE SERVINGS   **15 CALORIES PER SERVING**

1	C.	WATER
2	T.	HONEY
1	T.	ARROWROOT

1. Combine in a small sauce pan and cook and stir over low heat to thicken liquid. TO MICROWAVE: Combine in a glass 4 cup measuring cup and microwave 2 minutes on high. Remove and whisk. If mixture is not thick, microwave for another minute.

1/2	C.	RASPBERRY VINEGAR
1/2	T.	HAIN STONE GROUND MUSTARD

2. Combine and mix well.
3. Whisk into honey mixture and chill dressing.
4. Serve with mild greens and/or fresh fruit.

NOTE: Fruit vinegars are a wonderful way to add flavor to food without calories. Try this dressing on Bibb lettuce, orange slices and scallions—sensational!

SHEILA'S FITNESS TIP: To intensify a walking workout and burn more calories, make sure you're moving briskly. Every fourth step punch arms out in front or up into the air. Wear wrist weights if you're an old pro at punching.

CARB 4 GM (100%)   PROTEIN TRACE   FAT TRACE   SODIUM 8 MG

SOUR CREAM & VARIATIONS

MAKES 32 ONE TABLESPOON SERVINGS   **10 CALORIES PER SERVING**

1 1/2	C.	LOWFAT COTTAGE CHEESE (1%)
1/2	C.	BUTTERMILK
1	TSP.	FRESH LEMON JUICE

1. Combine in blender and process until smooth.
2. Store in refrigerator and serve in place of Sour Cream.

FOR TOASTED ONION DIP:

1/4	C.	ONION FLAKES, DRIED

1. Spread on a sheet of aluminum foil and place under broiler to brown.

1	T.	BERNARD JENSEN'S BROTH POWDER

2. Add to Sour Cream with Onion Flakes.
3. Serve with Potato Chips, Toasted Potato Skins or with a Baked Potato.

FOR TARTAR SAUCE:

2	T.	BELL PEPPER, DRIED
2	T.	ONION FLAKES, DRIED
1	TSP.	RED WINE VINEGAR

1. Add to Sour Cream and blend to just mix.
2. Serve with seafood.

NOTE: The calories in this are 75% lower than regular sour cream. This is a CALORIE SAVER TO KEEP ON HAND. Use it as you would any other Sour Cream.

SHEILA'S FITNESS TIPS: To stretch out your calves, stand about an arms distance from the wall, allow the upper body to come forward, keeping heels on the ground. Hold the stretch for 15 seconds; relax and repeat. If you wear high heels daily, this is a must!

CARB TRACE (21%)   **PROTEIN 1 GM. (65%)**   **FAT TRACE (14%)**   **SODIUM 47 MG.**

TAMARI TERIYAKI

MAKES 36 ONE TEASPOON SERVINGS   **2 CALORIES PER SERVING**

1/2	C.	TAMARI SOY SAUCE, LOW SODIUM
1 1/2	TSP.	HONEY
1	TSP.	FRESH GARLIC, MINCED
1/4	TSP.	FRESH GINGER, MINCED
2	T.	DRY SHERRY
1	T.	ONION, MINCED

1. Combine in a small pan and bring to a simmer.
2. Remove from heat immediately and cool.
3. Strain and use as a marinade for poultry or fish.

NOTE: This adds a lot of flavor to anything you want to put on your grill or cook over coals.

SHEILA'S FITNESS TIP: Muscles burn more calories than body fat of the same amount. Therefore, increase your muscle with upper body endurance training. You can use exercise machines at a fitness center or simply include push-ups in your personal exercise plan. Start with five, bent knee push-ups and work up to three sets of ten.

CARB TRACE (95%)   PROTEIN TRACE (5%)   FAT NONE   SODIUM 1 MG

THOUSAND ISLAND DRESSING

MAKES 32 ONE OUNCE SERVINGS   **20 CALORIES PER SERVING**

2	C.	TOMATO JUICE
1/2	C.	RED ONION, MINCED
1/4	C.	BELL PEPPER, MINCED

1. Combine in a sauce pan and simmer for 10 minutes.

2	T.	ARROWROOT
1/4	C.	TOMATO JUICE

2. Whisk together and stir into tomato mixture and cook and stir to thicken to a catsup consistency.
3. Chill.

2	C.	MAYONNAISE (FROM THIS CHAPTER OR COMMERCIAL LOWCAL)
2	T.	BALSAMIC VINEGAR
1/2	C.	PARSLEY, MINCED
1/2	C.	CHIVES, MINCED

4. Combine with tomato mixture and mix well.
5. Chill until ready to use.

NOTE: This is marvelous with seafood salads. You and your guests will never miss the fat and salt found in regular Thousand Island Dressings. If you absolutely must, add a little Pickle Relish, but it will add to the sugar and salt content.

SHEILA'S FITNESS TIP: To improve back flexibility, lie on the floor and pretend that you're being pulled in each direction from your hands above your head to your toes. Hold stretch for a count of 15, relax and repeat as often as you wish.

CARB 3 GM (99%)   **PROTEIN TRACE (1%)**   **FAT NONE**   **SODIUM TRACE**

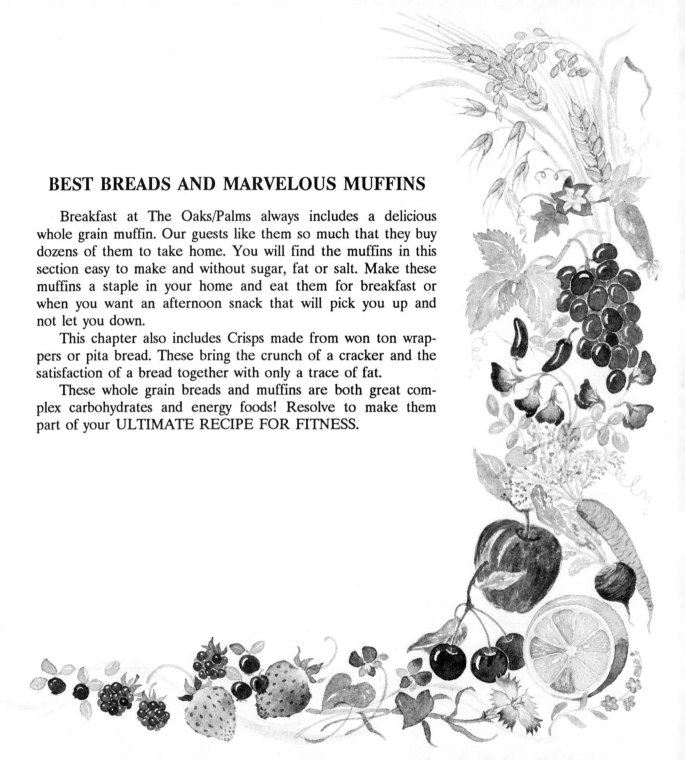

BEST BREADS AND MARVELOUS MUFFINS

Breakfast at The Oaks/Palms always includes a delicious whole grain muffin. Our guests like them so much that they buy dozens of them to take home. You will find the muffins in this section easy to make and without sugar, fat or salt. Make these muffins a staple in your home and eat them for breakfast or when you want an afternoon snack that will pick you up and not let you down.

This chapter also includes Crisps made from won ton wrappers or pita bread. These bring the crunch of a cracker and the satisfaction of a bread together with only a trace of fat.

These whole grain breads and muffins are both great complex carbohydrates and energy foods! Resolve to make them part of your ULTIMATE RECIPE FOR FITNESS.

APPLE DATE MUFFIN WITH WALNUTS

MAKES 30 MUFFINS   **65 CALORIES PER SERVING**

2		APPLES, PIPPIN OR GRANNY SMITH

1. Cut in quarters and chop coarsely in food processor.

2	C.	RAW WHEAT BRAN
1/3	C.	WHOLE WHEAT FLOUR
1	C.	APPLE JUICE CONCENTRATE
1/4	C.	DRY SHERRY
1	TSP.	VANILLA
1		EGG
2		EGG WHITES
1/2	C.	NONFAT YOGURT

2. Add to apples and process to mix well.

1	C.	ROLLED OATS
1	C.	DATES, CHOPPED
1/2	C.	WALNUTS, CHOPPED

3. Fold into apple mixture.
4. Set oven at 375 and spray a 10 inch cookie sheet with nonstick spray.
5. Form muffins, using your #24 scoop and bake for 25 to 30 minutes to brown.

NOTE: If you like sweets, you'll love this muffin! In fact you can make a lovely little drop cookie out of this recipe, too. Just don't tell the children it's good for them.

SHEILA'S FITNESS TIP: Do you know that stress can lower your immunity level? Beat stress with a regular, convenient and interesting workout or activity.

CARB 10 GM (63%)   **PROTEIN 2 GM (12%)**   **FAT 2 GM (25%)**   **SODIUM 7 MG**

APPLE NUT MUFFIN

MAKES 24 LARGE MUFFINS   **100 CALORIES PER SERVING**

3. C.   PIPPIN OR GRANNY SMITH APPLES, CORED AND QUARTERED
1 C.   CARROT, CUT

1. Place in food processor and process to chop coarsely.

1/2 C. OAT BRAN	**1 TSP. LOW SODIUM BAKING POWDER**
2 C. WHEAT BRAN	**1 TSP. BAKING SODA**
1 1/2 C. WHOLE WHEAT FLOUR	**2 TSP. CINNAMON**

2. Add to food processor, process to mix and transfer to a large mixing bowl.

1 EGG	**1/2 C. HONEY**
2 EGG WHITES	**3/4 C. WATER**
1 C. BUTTERMILK	

3. Place in food processor and process to whip.
4. Stir into the large mixing bowl.

1/2 C.   WALNUTS, CHOPPED

5. Fold into batter.
6. Line muffin tins with paper liners and spray liners with nonstick spray.
7. Form 24 muffins and bake at 350 for 50-55 minutes.

NOTE: This large and delicious muffin was developed at The Palms at Palm Springs and is a favorite with our guests. We like this as a late afternoon pick up with a cup of tea. This prevents an afternoon slump and takes us right up to dinner.

SHEILA'S FITNESS TIP: Best weight control tip of the day: Eat nothing while you're on your feet. Make sure that every time you eat, you are sitting at the table with your food on a dish. Many people are unaware of the calories that they consume while standing in front of the refrigerator and consume hundreds of calories that they don't really enjoy by 'just taking a little taste'. Then they wonder why they can't lose a few pounds.

CARB 16 MG (65%)   PROTEIN 3 GM (13%)   FAT 2 GM (21%)   SODIUM 21 MG

APPLESAUCE BRAN MUFFINS

MAKES 12 LARGE MUFFINS   **50 CALORIES PER SERVING**

2 C.	APPLES, CORED AND CUT	
1/4 C.	APPLE JUICE CONCENTRATE	OR 1 1/2 C. APPLE SAUCE

1. Combine and cook until apples are very tender. (This can be done in a sauce pan on the stove or in a glass cup in the microwave.)
2. Cool and process in food processor to applesauce consistency. Measure and use 1 1/2 C.

2   EGGS

3. Add to applesauce and process until mixture is whipped.

1 2/3 C.   WHEAT BRAN, UNPROCESSED
1/2 TSP.   BAKING POWDER, LOW SODIUM
1/2 TSP.   BAKING SODA
1/4 C.   POWDERED MILK (NONFAT)

4. Add to food processor and process to mix.
5. Spoon mixture into nonstick sprayed muffin tins and bake in a 375 oven for 30 minutes. (Press muffin with a finger. It should spring back when done rather than leaving an indentation.)
6. Remove from muffin tin and cool on a rack.

NOTE: This makes the lightest, largest low calorie muffin I have ever seen. It is sweet, moist and delicious. Add dried fruit and/or nuts as desired, remembering that the calories go up dramatically with these additions.

SHEILA'S FITNESS TIP: Avoid watching television while you're eating. Design dining time for pleasure by arranging your meals attractively on the plate. Choose a pretty napkin and treat yourself and your slimming body with respect.

CARB 5 GM (62%)   PROTEIN 3 GM (28%)   FAT 1 GM (27%)   SODIUM 20 MG

BANANA NUT MUFFIN

MAKES 16 LARGE MUFFINS   **65 CALORIES PER SERVING**

1 1/2	C.	MASHED BANANA
1		EGG
2		EGG WHITES

1. Combine in processor and process to whip. (Mixture will be light and fluffy.)

1 2/3	C.	WHEAT BRAN (RAW AND UNPROCESSED)
1/2	TSP.	LOW SODIUM BAKING POWDER
1/2	TSP.	BAKING SODA
1/4	C.	POWDERED MILK (NONFAT)

2. Add to banana mixture and mix well.

1/4	C.	WALNUTS OR PECANS, COARSELY CHOPPED

3. Fold into the batter and drop into 16 nonstick sprayed muffin cups.
4. Bake at 375 for a half an hour to brown and firm.
5. Remove immediately and cool on a rack.

NOTE: This can be converted into a BANANA RAISIN MUFFIN by substituting 1/2 cup raisins for the nuts. This change will save about 10 calories per muffin and lower the fat from 27% to a modest 17%.

SHEILA'S FITNESS TIP: If one is good, two has to be better, right? Not where socks and brisk walking or running are concerned because they constrict the feet too much. Try some of the newer acrylic socks which have proven to reduce the chance of blisters.

CARB 9 GM (56%)   PROTEIN 3 GM (17%)   FAT 2 GM (27%)   SODIUM 16 MG

BLUEBERRY MUFFIN

MAKES 24 MUFFINS   **55 CALORIES PER SERVING**

2	C.	WHEAT BRAN
1	C.	ROLLED OATS
1/4	C.	WHOLE WHEAT FLOUR
1	TSP.	CORIANDER

1. Combine in a large mixing bowl.

1		EGG
2		EGG WHITES
1/4	C.	HONEY
1	C.	NONFAT MILK

2. Combine, add to bran mixture and mix well.

2	C.	BLUEBERRIES
1/4	C.	GRAPENUTS

3. Add to batter and mix lightly to JUST combine.
4. Spray a cookie sheet with nonstick spray.
5. Form 24 muffins on a cookie sheet, using a #24 scoop.
6. Bake at 375 for 40 minutes to brown.

NOTE: Please feel free to use a different fruit or to use part oat bran. You can use nuts or seeds instead of the Grape Nuts or simply omit them. Nuts or seeds will bring the calorie content and percentage of fat higher. If you have no problem with cholesterol, it would be fine to use 2 whole eggs instead of 1 egg and 2 egg whites. It is FUN to create your own muffin recipes.

SHEILA'S FITNESS TIP: In a study of overweight women, it was found that those on a very low diet of 400 calories per day suffered muscle cell deterioration within two weeks. Muscles wouldn't contract and severe fatigue was the side effect. Keep your weight loss program balanced with foods such as the recipe above.

CARB 7 GM (66%)   PROTEIN 2 GM (22%)   FAT TRACE (12%)   SODIUM 20 MG

CARROT BREAD

MAKES 2 LOAVES (20 SLICES EACH)   **50 CALORIES PER SERVING**

2	C.	CARROTS, SHREDDED
3.	C.	WHOLE WHEAT FLOUR
1 1/2	TSP.	LOW SODIUM BAKING POWDER
1 1/2	TSP.	BAKING SODA
2	TSP.	CINNAMON
1	TSP.	CORIANDER

1. Combine in a large bowl and mix well.

2		EGG WHITES
1		EGG
2	C.	NONFAT MILK
1/4	C.	HONEY
1/4	C.	APPLE JUICE CONCENTRATE

2. Combine and mix with dry ingredients.
3. Divide between two nonstick sprayed loaf pans (8" x 4"). Or make 4 small loaves (3" x 6").
4. Bake at 350 for 50 to 60 minutes and turn bread out to cool on a rack.

NOTE: This is as good to eat as it is simple to make. It's a great feeling to have some of this in your freezer for lunch, brunch or afternoon tea. Try spreading it with some NONFAT YOGURT CREAM CHEESE and APPLE BUTTER ... delicious!

SHEILA'S FITNESS TIP: Do you realize that if you keep caffeine consumption to a minimum you might not crave snacks? Caffeine can increase nervousness, which in turn could make a weight watcher want to munch. Instead, drink diluted fruit juices, herbal teas and plenty of fresh and satisfying water.

CARB 11 GM (80%)   PROTEIN 2 GM (15%)   FAT TRACE (5%)   SODIUM 13 MG

CARROT RAISIN BRAN MUFFINS

MAKES 24 MUFFINS   **70 CALORIES PER SERVING**

1 C.	**RAISINS**	

1. Place in a glass measuring cup and cover with boiling water to soak, or heat in microwave to boiling.

1 C.	**BANANA**	1 C.	**CARROT PIECES**

2. Combine in food processor and process to grate carrot and mash banana.

2 1/2 C.	**WHEAT BRAN**	1/4 C.	**OAT BRAN**
1/2 C.	**RICE FLOUR**		

3. Add to banana mixture and process to mix.

1/2 C.	**APPLE JUICE CONCENTRATE**	1/2 C.	**NONFAT YOGURT**
1/2 C.	**WATER DRAINED FROM THE RAISINS**		

4. Add to food processor and mix well.

3/4 C.	**ROLLED OATS**	**THE SOAKED RAISINS**

5. Add to food processor and fold in with rubber spatula to distribute well without losing texture.
6. Spray a cookie sheet with nonstick spray and form 24 muffins on a cookie sheet, using a #24 scoop.
7. Bake at 375 for 45 minutes to brown the muffins.

NOTE: This is a CLEAN OUT THE REFRIGERATOR muffin that worked. Note that it is super low in fat and since I was out of eggs it has almost no cholesterol.

SHEILA'S FITNESS TIP: Do you know that you burn more calories cooking than bowling? For a 150 pound person, cooking uses about 3.5 calories per minute, while bowling burns 3.2 calories per minute. Neither can be considered aerobic but can add satisfaction and a social outlet to your regular fitness plan.

CARB 12 GM (79%)   PROTEIN 2 GM (14%)   FAT TRACE (7%)   SODIUM 7 MG

CINNAMON APPLE PECAN ROLLS

MAKES 24 LARGE ROLLS   **90 CALORIES PER SERVING**

1	T.	BAKERS YEAST
1/3	C.	WARM WATER

1 TSP. HONEY

1. Combine in food processor and set aside to allow the yeast to activate.

2 1/2	C.	WHOLE WHEAT FLOUR
1	C.	WARM WATER

1 T.   BLACK STRAP MOLASSES

2. Add to yeast mixture and process the mixture until it forms a ball.
3. Turn the dough out on a lightly floured bread board.
4. Using your floured hands or a rolling pin, flatten dough into a 10" x 12" rectangle .

1/4	C.	CONCENTRATED APPLE JUICE
2	T.	HONEY

1 TSP. CINNAMON

5. Combine and mix well.

3.	C.	SLICED APPLE

1 T.   WHOLE WHEAT FLOUR

6. Toss together and then add enough of the apple juice mixture to moisten, reserving leftover juice.
7. Spread apple mixture over the of dough, roll and slice into 24 pieces.
8. Set rolls on their sides on a nonstick sprayed cookie sheet and paint with reserved juice.

1/4	C.	TOASTED PECAN PIECES

9. Sprinkle Cinnamon Rolls with pecans and cover loosely with a piece of plastic wrap and set in a warm place for 30 minutes to allow dough to rise.
10. Remove the plastic and bake at 350 for 30 minutes to brown the rolls.
11. Serve to your favorite people for breakfast along with some fresh fruit and yogurt.

NOTE: Wait until your friends and family discover that they can have these wonderfully sweet and crunchy rolls as part of Spa Cuisine. They'll love it!

CARB 21 GM (75)   PROTEIN 2 GM (9%)   FAT 2 GM (16%)   SODIUM 3 MG

CORNMEAL MUFFIN

MAKES 24 MUFFINS   **60 CALORIES PER SERVING**

2	C.	YELLOW CORNMEAL

1. Place in food processor and process with steel blade to produce a lighter texture.

1	C.	BUTTERMILK
1 1/4	C.	SKIM MILK
2	T.	HONEY
1		EGG YOLK

2. Add to food processor and process to mix well.

4		EGG WHITES

3. Place in a large bowl and whip until stiff but not dry.
4. FOLD cornmeal mixture into whipped egg whites. Do this
with a light hand to maintain as much air as possible for volume.
5. Line muffin tins with paper liners and spray liners with nonstick spray.
Prepare 24 paper liners.
6. Spoon a heaping tablespoon of batter into each liner.
7. Bake at 350 for 20 minutes to brown the muffins.

NOTE: Cornmeal combines with beans to produce a complete protein. Mexicans know what they are doing when they serve Corn Tortillas with beans . . . and they taste so good together. For a JALAPENO CORNMEAL MUFFIN, fold a tablespoon or two of Jalapeno peppers into the batter right before forming the muffins . . . and if you also add 1/4 cup of grated cheese, I think you'll be pleased with the results.

SHEILA'S FITNESS TIP: Golf or tennis your sport? Here's a stretch you need. Grasp an elbow with the opposite hand, pull the elbow across your body, hold for fifteen seconds, release and repeat five times on each shoulder.

CARB 2 GM (77%)   PROTEIN 2 GM (16%)   FAT 1 GM (8%)   SODIUM 27 MG

CRANBERRY WHEAT GERM MUFFIN

MAKES 12 MUFFINS   **110 CALORIES PER SERVING**

1 1/3 C.   WHOLE WHEAT FLOUR
  1/3 C.   WHEAT GERM
    1 T.   BAKING POWDER, LOW SODIUM
            1. Combine in a large mixing bowl.

  3/4 C.   NONFAT MILK
    1   EGG WHITE, BEATEN
    2 T.   CANOLA OIL
  1/3 C.   HONEY
            2. Combine and mix well.
            3. Add to dry ingredients, mixing until just combined.

    1 C.   CRANBERRIES, FRESH OR FROZEN (OR BLUEBERRIES)
            4. Fold into batter and then fill 12 nonstick coated muffin cups ... or line muffin
cups with papers.
            5. Bake at 375 for 25 minutes to brown.

NOTE: This is more like a traditional muffin than most of our heavy food processor mixed muffins. However, its a nice change, quite simple to do and wonderful to eat!

SHEILA'S FITNESS TIP: Love to walk, but not alone? Mall walkers are everywhere. Contact your local shopping center for a mall walking club or start your own. Most mall walkers exercise before the stores open. The environment is controlled and security guards are normally within sight.

CARB 19 GM (66%)   PROTEIN 3 GM (12%)   FAT 3 GM (23%)   SODIUM 18 MG

CREPES (SUPER LOW FAT)

MAKES 8 CREPES   **15 CALORIES PER SERVING**

1/2	C.	NONFAT MILK
2	T.	POWDERED MILK (NONFAT)
4		EGG WHITES

1. Combine in a bowl and whisk to mix.
2. Coat crepe pan with nonstick spray and heat on low until hot (Sizzle a drop of water).
3. Add 1 ounce of crepe mixture and tilt pan to distribute batter evenly over the entire bottom of pan.
4. Cook over low heat until firm.
5. Place under broiler to brown top OR remove and fill crepe.

NOTE: You will find many recipes which use these crepes in this book, especially in the VEGIE MAIN DISH SECTION. Using just egg whites rather than the whole egg took the fat percentage from a large 56% to a tiny 2%. If you choose to use one egg and two egg whites, the calories go to 30 per crepe and the percentage of fat to 23. I do prefer the taste of the crepe using just one whole egg, but if I had high cholesterol, I would use just egg whites. These crepes freeze well.

SHEILA'S FITNESS TIP: Confused about all the cholesterol controversy? Here are some tips: Have your cholesterol level tested, reduce all fats in your diet, exercise regularly and stop smoking. Oat bran is included in the scrumptious muffins served at The Oaks and The Palms but you can also sprinkle oat bran into soups, cereals, blender drinks and on top of salads for healthful affects.

CARB 1 GM (30%)   PROTEIN 2 GM (68%)   FAT TRACE (2%)   SODIUM 33 MG

DESERT DATE MUFFIN

MAKES 12 MUFFINS   **90 CALORIES PER SERVING**

1	C.	CARROTS, CUT

1. Place in food processor to chop fine.

2		EGG WHITES
1		EGG
1	C.	BUTTERMILK
2	T.	BLACKSTRAP MOLASSES

2. Add to carrots and process to mix well.

2 1/2	C.	WHEAT BRAN
1/2	C.	WHEAT GERM
2	TSP.	CINNAMON

3. Add to carrot mixture and mix well.

1/2	C.	DATES, CHOPPED

4. Fold into batter.
5. Form muffins by heaping into a #24 scoop and dropping on a nonstick sprayed cookie sheet.
6. Bake at 375 for about 25 minutes or until brown.

NOTE: This is a revised version of a muffin developed to celebrate the opening of The Palms at Palm Springs. The cooks at The Oaks tell me that it is our third most popular muffin. We can tell because most of our guests become so addicted to a muffin for breakfast that they order their favorites to take home.

SHEILA'S FITNESS TIP: Stay away from long term goals when it comes to fitness and weight control. Instead make mini-goals and you'll see results . . . one successful week at a time.

CARB 13 GM (60%)   PROTEIN 5 GM (23%)   FAT 2 GM (18%)   SODIUM 43 MG

GLAMOUR MUFFIN

MAKES 24 MUFFINS   **60 CALORIES PER SERVING**

2		PIPPIN OR GRANNY SMITH APPLES

1. Cut apples in about 8 pieces. Do not peel or core.
2. Place apple in food processor and process to chop coarsely.

2	C.	WHEAT BRAN, RAW OR UNPROCESSED
1/4	C.	WHOLE WHEAT FLOUR
2	TSP.	CINNAMON
1	TSP.	NUTMEG
2		EGG WHITES
1		EGG
1	C.	BUTTERMILK
1/4	C.	BLACKSTRAP MOLASSES

3. Add to food processor and process to mix well.

1	C.	ROLLED OATS
1/4	C.	SUNFLOWER SEEDS

4. Add and process to just mix, taking care not to lose the texture of the oats and seeds.
5. Using a #24 scoop, form muffins on a nonstick sprayed cookie sheet.
6. Bake at 375 for 40 minutes to brown.

NOTE: This muffin was developed for a feature done on our food at The Palms at Palm Springs by *Glamour Magazine*. This is a revised version of the original. By dropping one egg yolk and substituting two egg whites I was able to get the fat under 30% and the taste is just as good.

SHEILA'S FITNESS TIP: Dining out? Plan what you are going to eat *before* entering the restaurant.

CARB 6 GM (51%)   PROTEIN 3 GM (22%)   FAT 1 GM (27%)   SODIUM 22 MG

ONION ROLLS OR BREADSTICKS

MAKES 40 ROLLS OR BREADSTICKS   **70 CALORIES PER SERVING**

5 C.   WHOLE WHEAT FLOUR
1. Place in a bowl and heat in a 350 oven to heat through.

1/2 C.   DRIED ONION FLAKES   **2 T.   LOW SODIUM SOY SAUCE**
2. Combine, mix well and set aside.

1 C.   WARM WATER

2 T.   BAKERS YEAST
1 T.   HONEY
3. Combine in food processor and set aside to allow the yeast to activate.

1 1/2 C.   WARM WATER   **2 T.   BLACK STRAP MOLASSES**
4. Combine and add to yeast mixture with the warmed flour and onion mixture.
5. Process to mix well, then run processor until the dough forms a ball.

1/4 C.   WHOLE WHEAT FLOUR   **2 T.   POPPY, CHIA OR SESAME SEEDS**
6. Flour a bread board and turn dough out on board.
7. Knead until enough flour is absorbed so that dough is not sticky and can be handled.
8. Pat dough out with hands, sprinkle with seeds and divide into 40 pieces, forming rolls or breadsticks as desired.
9. Place on a nonstick sprayed cookie sheet in a warm spot to rise.
10. When rolls have almost doubled in size, bake at 350 for 30 minutes to brown.
11. Serve to delighted guests and family.

NOTE: Try making half of this recipe into a loaf and the other half into 20 rolls or breadsticks. Roll them in poppy seeds and grated parmesan cheese... This makes them super special!

SHEILA'S FITNESS TIP: In a restaurant, don't send the bread away — get rid of the butter!

CARB 13 GM (72%)   PROTEIN 3 GM (14%)   FAT 1 GM (13%)   SODIUM 3 MG

ONION SWISS TURNOVERS

2 OZ. JARLSBURG SWISS CHEESE
3/4 C. LOWFAT COTTAGE CHEESE (1%)
  1. Place Swiss Cheese in food processor and process.
  2. Add Cottage Cheese, process smooth and set aside.

1 C. RED ONION, COARSELY CHOPPED
  4. Fold into cheese mixture.

1 EGG WHITE, LIGHTLY BEATEN WITH A FORK
1 T. PARMESAN CHEESE, GRATED
  5. Prepare and set aside.

4 FILLO DOUGH SHEETS
  6. Thaw according to package directions and lay out two sheets, stacked on top of each other.
  7. Start one inch down from the top and spread 1/4 cup of cheese mixture in a strip across the sheet.
  8. Roll fillo Dough over jelly roll style, stopping half way down the sheet.
  9. Cut the sheet across and seal with egg white.
  10. Place roll on a nonstick sprayed cookie sheet, paint the top with egg white and sprinkle with Parmesan Cheese.
  11. Using kitchen scissors, cut roll into 10 pieces.
  12. Repeat this operation and bake in a 400 degree oven for 15 minutes.

NOTE: These freeze well and will be hot and crisp after 7 minutes in a 450 oven.

SHEILA'S FITNESS TIP: Walking a 17 minute mile uses about 5.4 calories per minute.

CARB 2 GM (48%)   PROTEIN 1 GM (37%)   FAT TRACE (15%)   SODIUM 29 MG.

ORANGE OAT MUFFIN

MAKES 18 MUFFINS   **95 CALORIES PER SERVING**

2	C.	CARROTS, CUT

1. Place in food processor and process to chop fine.

1/4	C.	BROWN RICE FLOUR
1/4	TSP.	CORIANDER
1	C.	ORANGE JUICE
1		EGG
2		EGG WHITES
1	TSP.	VANILLA

2. Add to food processor and process to mix.

3 1/2	C.	ROLLED OATS
1/2	C.	DATES, CHOPPED

3. Fold into batter.
4. Form muffins on a nonstick sprayed cookie sheet, using 1/4 cup measure or a heaping # 24 scoop.
5. Bake at 350 for 50 minutes or until brown.

NOTE: If you have an allergy to wheat or milk, this muffin was designed with you in mind. However, it tastes so good that your nonallergic friends will want some, too. Try dropping the batter by teaspoons, flattening with a fork and baking as a cookie. It is fantastic topped with a bit of NONFAT YOGURT CREAM CHEESE and ORANGE MARMALADE. Both recipes are in DRESSINGS, DIPS AND SPREADS.

SHEILA'S FITNESS TIP: If you run or walk at night, take along some light. Use hand held flashlights as weights and also make yourself more visible. Shine one to the front and one to the rear.

CARB 8 GM (60%)   **PROTEIN 3 GM (26%)**   **FAT 1 GM (15%)**   **SODIUM 13 MG**

PARMESAN PITA CRISPS

MAKES 24 TWO PIECE SERVINGS   **30 CALORIES PER SERVING**

6   **MINI WHOLE WHEAT PITAS**
1. Cut into quarters and split.
2. Lay rough side up on a cookie sheet, close together.

2 T.   **PARMESAN CHEESE, GRATED**
3. Sprinkle cheese over pita pieces and bake at 350 for 10 minutes to brown and crisp.
4. Serve as a bread or cracker with soup or salad.

NOTE: For those of us who enjoy bread but like to watch our fat calories, these are superb. They have so much flavor and crunch that no one feels the need to add butter. If you choose to cut the pitas into sixths, the calories go down to 10 per crisp. We sometimes skip the Parmesan and use the resulting crackers as chips for dips.

SHEILA'S FITNESS TIP: Firm the inner thighs: Lying on your back on an exercise mat, press a sofa pillow between your knees as you contract your abdominal muscles. Hold for a count of ten, release and repeat for a total of ten times.

CARB 6 GM (73%)   **PROTEIN 1 GM (17%)**   **FAT TRACE (10%)**   **SODIUM 20 MG**

POPOVERS

3/4 C.   WHOLE WHEAT PASTRY FLOUR
1/4 C.   BROWN RICE FLOUR
1. Sift before measuring and place in a 400 degree oven to heat. (Leave oven 'on' to bake popovers.)

2   EGGS
2   EGG WHITES
2. Place in a large bowl and whip with electric mixer until thick.

1 1/2 C.   NONFAT MILK
1 TSP. HONEY
1 TSP. CANOLA OIL
3. Combine in blender with warmed flour and process to blend well.
4. With electric mixer running, add flour mixture to eggs.
5. Spray muffin tins with nonstick spray. (1/2 cup size)
6. Fill tins half full, keeping batter well stirred.
7. Bake in 400 degree oven for 20 minutes. Turn oven off and leave for 15 minutes.
8. With a small sharp knife, make a slit in each Popover.
9. Serve with honey, APPLE BUTTER or ORANGE MARMALADE.

NOTE: These will turn any meal into a party. Be sure to use a light hand in measuring the flour so that your POPOVERS will really pop! We also serve these for dessert filled with WHIPPED CREAM, GLAZED FRUIT or puddings.

SHEILA'S FITNESS TIP: Do you want to know how to look like you've just lost five pounds? Stand, sit, walk tall and check your posture regularly. Besides looking thinner, good posture promotes healthy organ function.

CARB 5 GM (56%)   PROTEIN 2 GM (23%)   FAT 1 GM (21%)   SODIUM 18 MG

SPOON BREAD TOPPING

| 1 1/2 | C. | NONFAT MILK |
| 1 | T. | BUTTER BUDS |

1. Combine in a sauce pan and heat to just below boiling. TO MICROWAVE: Combine in a glass 4 cup measuring cup and microwave 3 minutes to heat milk.

| 1/2 | C. | YELLOW CORN MEAL |

2. Whisk into milk, heat and stir on low to thicken mixture. TO MICROWAVE: Whisk into milk, microwave 2 minutes and whisk again.

4	OZ.	(LIFETIME) MOZZARELLA AND CHEDDAR CHEESE
1		EGG
3		EGG WHITES

3. Combine in food processor to chop cheese and mix.
4. With processor running, add corn meal mixture and mix well.
5. Pour over any hot casserole mixture and bake at 375 for 30 minutes to brown.

NOTE: This is marvelous as a topping for the TAMALE PIE or CHILE but it can take any ordinary casserole dish and make it look and taste quite extraordinary.

SHEILA'S FITNESS TIP: Stimulate healthy skin with a facial mask. While this recipe is cooking, mix equal amounts of yogurt and honey and smooth it on your clean face. Wait fifteen minutes and rinse well. Apply a moisturizer that includes a sun screen.

CARB 10 GM (42%)   PROTEIN 9 GM (40%)   FAT 2 GM (18%)   SODIUM 76 MG

TRIPLE APPLE OAT BRAN MUFFIN

MAKES 30 MUFFINS   **75 CALORIES PER SERVING**

1/2 C.   **RAISINS**
           1. Place in measuring cup and cover with boiling water.
           2. Set aside to plump raisins.

2 MED. **PIPPIN OR GRANNY SMITH APPLES**
           3. Wash, quarter and process in food processor to chop coarsely.

2 C.   **OAT BRAN**   2   **EGG WHITES**
1/3 C.   **BROWN RICE FLOUR**   1 C.   **NONFAT YOGURT**
1 TSP.   **CINNAMON**   1 C.   **APPLE JUICE CONCENTRATE**
1/2 TSP. **CORIANDER**
           4. Add to apples and process to mix well.

1 1/2 C. **ROLLED OATS (NOT INSTANT)**
1/2 C.   **GRAPE NUTS**
           THE PLUMPED RAISINS, DRAINED
           5. Add to apple mixture and process just enough to mix. Take care not to
           over mix and lose texture.
           6. Form muffins using a #24 scoop and place on a non-stick cookie sheet.
           7. Bake at 375 for 25 to 30 minutes to brown.

NOTE: Both the apple and the oat bran are said to lower cholesterol so these are a fine breakfast
for anyone with high cholesterol...besides, they taste wonderful!

SHEILA'S FITNESS TIP: In a recent survey, 37 percent of those polled say they exercise to
increase self esteem, 32 percent to reduce blood pressure, 23 percent to decrease cholesterol, 14
percent to lessen diabetic symptoms and 11 percent to increase energy. However, 100 percent soon
find that exercise can do all those things and make you feel great while you're working out.

CARB 12 GM (73%)   PROTEIN 3 GM (18%)   FAT 1 GM (9%)   SODIUM 21 GM

WON TON CRISPS

MAKES 6 SERVINGS OF 2 EACH   **6 CALORIES PER SERVING**

12   WON TON SKINS
            1. Cut in half diagonally and lay on a cookie sheet.

1 TSP. LOW SODIUM SOY SAUCE
            2. Paint Won Tons with soy sauce using a pastry brush.

1 TSP. SESAME SEEDS (OPTIONAL)
            3. Sprinkle on Won Tons and bake at 375 for 6 to 8 minutes to brown.
            4. Set aside to cool and serve as a cracker with Oriental food.

NOTE: We sometimes serve this with a FRUIT SOUP (recipe in Soup Section), but we change the flavor by painting the Won Tons with apple juice concentrate before baking. I have served them with CRAB SALAD to my bridge foursome with very happy results.

SHEILA'S FITNESS TIP: Making slim food choices will result in a slimmer you—1/2 grapefruit instead of 1/2 avocado saves 120 calories, 5 dates rather than 5 dried figs saves 125 calories and 1/2 cup of evaporated skim milk rather than cream will save you 320 calories.

CARB 1 GM (79%)   **PROTEIN TRACE (2%)**   **FAT TRACE (20%)**   **SODIUM 12 MG**

SENSATIONAL SOUPS

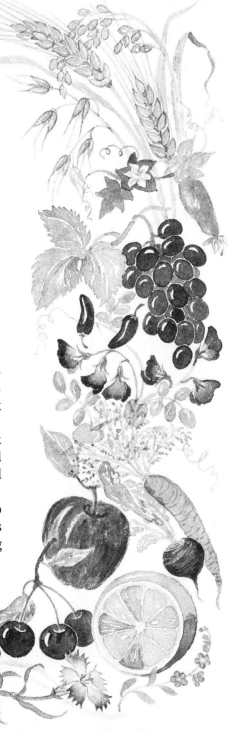

Soups can make a hearty meal with some delicious whole grain bread and a mixed green salad. The Cioppino, Bean Soups, Clam Chowder, Poultry Soups and Minestrone all fall into that category. When you determine which ones are your favorites, make them in your largest kettle and freeze individual portions in soup mugs or bowls. Soups are real comfort foods especially when you have your favorites waiting in your freezer for the nights you are too busy or too tired to cook!

You'll also find cool soups to use as a first course. The Fresh Fruit Soup, a Spa favorite, is so easy you'll make it often.

We have included some wonderful soups made from vegetables only. Use them to start a meal or serve with a sandwich as the whole meal.

If you have a favorite soup that is high in fat, with cream as a base and butter as its main seasoning, you don't have to give it up. You can decalorize it. Substitute Evaporated Skim Milk for the cream and season with Butter Buds.

You can also leave the salt out of all soups. We use a lot of Bernard Jensen's Broth Powder and herbs, both fresh and dried. Most soups are improved with a sprinkle of fresh snipped parsley and chives.

Countless studies have been done showing that people who eat soup lose weight. Since warm liquid is filling and soup is mostly water, it makes sense. You might decide to make eating more soups part of your ULTIMATE RECIPE FOR FITNESS.

BLACK BEAN SOUP

2 C. **BLACK BEANS**   1 1/2 QT. **WATER**

1. Rinse beans, place in kettle with water and bring to a boil.
2. Boil for 2 minutes, remove from heat and soak for at least 1 hour or overnight.
3. Drain and rinse beans.

2 QT. **WATER**   2 **BAY LEAVES**
3 T. **BERNARD JENSEN'S BROTH POWDER**

4. Combine with beans, bring to a boil and simmer for 2 hours or until beans are tender.

1 C. **ONION, MINCED**   1 C. **CELERY, CHOPPED**
1 T. **GARLIC, MINCED**   1 TSP. **OREGANO**
1 C. **BELL PEPPER, CHOPPED**   1 TSP. **CUMIN**

5. Add to beans during last hour of cooking.
6. When beans are tender, remove 1/2 to blender or food processor and puree. Let cool before processing.
7. Stir pureed beans into kettle and reheat.

1/4 C. **CREAMY CHEESE (see DRESSINGS, DIPS AND SPREADS) Or**
1/4 C. **LOWFAT MOZZARELLA, GRATED**
1/4 C. **CHIVES OR SCALLIONS, SNIPPED**

8. Serve the soup in heated bowls and top with 1 tsp. of cheese and a sprinkle of chives.

NOTE: This makes a wonderful meal accompanied by a big TOSSED GREEN SALAD. This soup can also be served chilled with Lowcal Sour Cream instead of the cheese.

CARB 14 GM (52%)   PROTEIN 10 GM (37%)   FAT 1 GM (11%)   SODIUM 80 MG

CIOPPINO (ITALIAN FISH CHOWDER)

MAKES 6 SERVINGS   **150 CALORIES PER SERVING**

3 C.   TOMATO JUICE
        1. Place in a kettle and bring to a simmer.

1/2 C.   ONION, CHOPPED   1/4 TSP.   MARJORAM
1/2 C.   CELERY, SLICED THIN   1/4 TSP.   OREGANO
1 TSP.   GARLIC POWDER   1/2 LB.   FRESH FISH, BONED
1/4 TSP. ROSEMARY
        2. Add to kettle and simmer for an hour to thicken broth.

1 C.   FRESH MUSHROOMS, SLICED   6   CLAMS IN THE SHELL
1/4 C.   RED WINE   1/2 LB.   FISH CHUNKS, BITE SIZED
6 LG.   SHRIMP IN THE SHELL
        3. Add to kettle and reheat. The seafood listed above may be cooked or raw. If it is
        raw, simmer until the seafood is just cooked. If the seafood is cooked, simmer briefly
        to cook the mushrooms.

2 T.   PARMESAN CHEESE, GRATED   6   PARSLEY SPRIGS
6   LEMON WEDGES
        4. Serve the Cioppino in heated bowls, topped with a sprinkle of cheese, a wedge of
        lemon and a sprig of parsley.

NOTE: This is a revised version of an old Oaks/Palms favorite. It is an excellent way to use left over fish, and even folks who are not fond of seafood like it. Since few people eat the recommended two to three servings of fish per week, give this recipe a try and increase your weekly seafood consumption.

SHEILA'S FITNESS TIP: If you weigh 150 lbs. and walk for 40 minutes, you will burn off approximately 150 calories — one entire serving of Cioppino.

CARB 8 GM (24%)   PROTEIN 24 GM (66%)   FAT 2 GM (10%)   SODIUM 546 MG

CLAM CHOWDER

MAKES 6 ONE CUP SERVINGS   130 CALORIES PER SERVING

2 C.   POTATOES, SCRUBBED   2 C.   ONION, MINCED
       AND CUBED   2 1/2 C.   CHICKEN STOCK, BOILING
2 C.   CAULIFLOWER, CUBED

1. Combine in a soup pot and cook 15 minutes until potatoes are tender.
2. Remove from heat and mash, leaving some chunks.

1/2 T.   ONION POWDER   1/2 TSP.   MARJORAM
1/2 T.   DILL WEED

3. Grind together in mortar and pestle and add to pot.

2 T.   ARROWROOT   1/3 C.   WATER
1 T.   BERNARD JENSEN'S BROTH POWDER

4. Combine, whisk together and stir into soup.
5. Heat and stir to thicken broth.

1 C.   BUTTERMILK
10 OZ. CLAM MEAT, FRESH OR FROZEN PREFERRED

6. Add and reheat.

2 T.   CHIVES OR SCALLIONS, SNIPPED

7. Serve the soup in heated bowls and top with a sprinkle of chives.

NOTE: This is a favorite soup we serve with a sandwich for lunch at The Oaks. We melt a bit of Lifetime Cheese on a slice of our wonderful whole grain bread, top it with a slice of tomato and some Italian Herbs and have a very satisfying meal.

SHEILA'S FITNESS TIP: If you're bored with one form of exercise, try cross-training, run, walk, cycle and swim. Vary your workout and you will find it easier to stay motivated.

CARB 18 GM (58%)   PROTEIN 10 GM (33%)   FAT 1 GM (9%)   SODIUM 34 MG

COSTA RICAN TOMATO SOUP

MAKES 6 SERVINGS   **30 CALORIES PER SERVING**

2 1/2	C.	TOMATO JUICE, UNSALTED

1. Place in sauce pan and bring to a simmer.

1/2	C.	CARROT, GRATED
2	T.	CELERY, MINCED
2	T.	CHIVES, MINCED
3	T.	ONION, MINCED
2	T.	GREEN BELL PEPPER, MINCED BASIL
1/8	TSP.	BLACK PEPPER, GROUND
1/4	TSP.	HONEY

2. Add to tomato juice and simmer for 30 minutes until all vegetables are cooked.

2	T.	FRESH PARSLEY, MINCED
1/3	C.	BUTTERMILK

3. Add to the soup and return to a simmer. Do not allow soup to boil after adding milk.

4. Serve in heated bowls and garnish with a sprinkle of fresh parsley.

NOTE: This has an unusual but delicious flavor. It is a frequently requested recipe by our spa guests ... and a great beginning to any meal.

SHEILA'S FITNESS TIP: Remember, to experience the physical benefits of exercise, you will need to be consistent: 3 times a week, for 12 weeks. The emotional benefits may surface immediately.

CARB 6 GM (76%)   PROTEIN 1 GM (18%)   FAT TRACE (6%)   SODIUM 60 MG

CRAB SOUP WITH SAFFRON RICE

MAKES 6 SERVINGS   100 CALORIES PER SERVING

2/3	C.	BROWN RICE
1/2	TSP.	SAFFRON
1 1/3	C.	WATER

1. Bring water to a boil, add rice and saffron, cover and heat on low for 1 hour or until all water is absorbed.

1	QT.	CHICKEN BROTH OR STOCK
1	C.	CRAB MEAT, SHREDDED
		THE COOKED RICE

2. Heat together and serve in heated bowls.

| 1 | T. | FRESH PARSLEY, MINCED (OR CILANTRO IF YOU LIKE IT) |

3. Garnish with the parsley.

NOTE: This is a simple way to use left over rice and crab. It was developed by David Del Nagro, Oaks Head Chef by way of the famous Ranch House Restaurant. His recipe calls for cilantro, which I dislike, so I substitute parsley.

SHEILA'S FITNESS TIP: If you are a person who finds it difficult to make time to exercise for 30 minutes, try 3 ten-minute exercise breaks. Current research indicates that you get almost the same fitness benefit.

CARB 8 MG (64%)   PROTEIN 3 GM (26%)   FAT 1 GM (11%)   SODIUM 90 MG

CREAM OF CARROT SOUP

MAKES 12 SERVINGS   **35 CALORIES PER SERVING**

| 3 | C. | WATER |
| 1 | T. | BERNARD JENSEN'S BROTH POWDER |

1. Combine in sauce pan and bring to a boil.

| 4 1/2 | C. | CARROTS, CUT IN PIECES | 1/2 | C. | CELERY, CHOPPED |
| 1 1/2 | C. | ONION, CHOPPED | 1 | | BAY LEAF |

2. Add to boiling water, reduce to a simmer and cook until carrots are tender.
3. Remove bay leaf and cool.

| 1 | TSP. | CURRY POWDER |
| 1 1/2 | C. | WATER |

4. Place carrot mixture in blender and puree with curry powder, adding water as needed to form a thick soup.
5. Return soup to pan and reheat.

| 1 | C. | BUTTERMILK |
| 1 1/2 | T. | CORNSTARCH |

6. Stir into soup and reheat without boiling.

| 2 | T. | CHIVES, MINCED |

7. Serve soup in heated bowls topped with a sprinkle of chives.

NOTE: This is also delicious served chilled. Carrots are one of the best sources of Beta Carotene so this would be a splendid addition to your repertoire of recipes. (Beta Carotene helps build a strong immune system.)

SHEILA'S FITNESS TIP: Don't skip meals in your effort to lose weight. Eating raises your metabolism which helps to burn calories.

CARB 7 GM (77%)   **PROTEIN 1 GM (15%)**   **FAT TRACE (8%)**   **SODIUM 41 MG**

CREAM OF CAULIFLOWER SOUP

3 C.   CAULIFLOWER, CUT IN SMALL PIECES
1. Steam or microwave until tender and cool (or use left-over cooked cauliflower).

1/2 C.   LOWFAT COTTAGE CHEESE (1%)
1 T.   NONFAT YOGURT
1 T.   PARMESAN CHEESE, GRATED
2 TSP.   BERNARD JENSEN'S BROTH POWDER
1/8 TSP.   DRIED DILL WEED
2. Combine in food processor and process smooth.
3. Add cauliflower and process to a smooth puree.

2 C.   NONFAT MILK
4. Slowly add one cup of milk to food processor contents. When mixture liquefies, pour it into a sauce pan and add the rest of the milk.
5. Heat and stir over low heat until hot but not boiling.

2 T.   CHIVES OR SCALLIONS, MINCED
1 TSP.   PAPRIKA
2 T.   PARMESAN CHEESE, GRATED
6. Serve in heated bowls topped with the above.

NOTE: You could, of course, heat the soup one cup at a time in your microwave. This is especially helpful for small families. Freeze or refrigerate the remainder in soup cups.

SHEILA'S FITNESS TIPS: Medium-intensity aerobics to music can be great fun and a super way to develop energy and stamina. The heavier you are, the more calories you will burn per minute. A 115 to 125 lb. person burns approximately 370 calories per hour, but if you are 180 to 190 lbs. you burn 520 calories per hour.

CARB 8 GM (45%)   PROTEIN 8 GM (41%)   FAT 1 GM (14%)   SODIUM 180 MG

CURRIED CHICKEN SOUP

MAKES 12 SERVINGS   **120 CALORIES PER SERVING**

2	TSP.	PEANUT OIL	2	TSP.	GARLIC, MINCED
1	C.	ONION, CHOPPED	2	TSP.	FRESH GINGER, MINCED

1. Heat oil in soup kettle and saute onion, garlic and ginger until tender.

2	TSP.	CURRY POWDER	1	TSP.	TUMERIC
1	T.	BROTH POWDER	1	TSP.	ALLSPICE

2. Add to kettle and stir into onion mixture.

1/2	C.	TOMATO PASTE	1 1/2	C.	WATER

3. Add to kettle and bring to a boil.

2	C.	GREEN BEANS, CUT	3	C.	CAULIFLOWER, CUT
2	C.	CARROTS, SLICED THIN	3	C.	NONFAT MILK

4. Add to kettle, return to a simmer and cook for 30 minutes
until vegetables are tender.

1/4	C.	ARROWROOT	1/2	C.	NONFAT MILK

5. Combine, whisk smooth and stir into soup to thicken.

1/2	LB.	CHICKEN, COOKED AND SHREDDED

6. Add to soup and reheat.

1/4	C.	NONFAT YOGURT	2	T.	SCALLIONS, MINCED
1/4	C.	APPLE, MINCED			

7. Serve soup in heated bowls, top with a dollop of yogurt, apple and scallions.

NOTE: A curry lovers delight!

CARB 4 GM (27%)   PROTEIN 8 GM (62%)   FAT TRACE (10%)   SODIUM 20 MG

EGG DROP SOUP WITH TOFU

MAKES 12 SERVINGS   **20 CALORIES PER SERVING**

NONSTICK SPRAY
> 1. Spray sauce pan and heat.

1	TSP.	SOY SAUCE, LOW SODIUM
3/4	C.	ONION, MINCED
1	TSP.	GARLIC, MINCED
1/2	C.	CELERY, DICED

> 2. Combine in sauce pan and saute 2-3 minutes.

1 1/2 C.   POULTRY STOCK OR WATER AND BROTH POWDER (2 TSP.)
> 2. Add to onion mixture and simmer for 30 minutes.

2   EGG WHITES, BEATEN
> 3. Bring soup to a hard boil, stir in egg whites and remove from heat.

1/2 LB.   TOFU, DRAINED
> 4. Press out all possible liquid and slice thin to resemble noodles.
> 5. Add to soup and reheat.

1/2 C.   SCALLIONS, SLICED VERY THIN
> 6. Serve soup in heated bowls and top with a sprinkle of scallions.

NOTE: This has been a popular soup at The Oaks/Palms for years. By taking out the egg yolks and adding tofu, we have a better soup that is much lower in fat than the original. Why don't you see how much fat and cholesterol you can get out of some of your old recipes?

> SHEILA'S FITNESS TIP: Set a realistic goal for your body. Know that your fitness and food plan can help you make positive changes but will not take fat off of specific areas or make a five foot person six feet tall.

CARB 1 GM (16%)   PROTEIN 3 GM (52%)   FAT 1 GM (31%)   SODIUM 95 MG

FRESH FRUIT SOUP

MAKES 6 SERVINGS   **45 CALORIES PER SERVING**

1 1/2 C.   MASHED FRESH FRUIT (STRAWBERRIES, PEACHES, MELON, MANGO, PAPAYA, ETC.)
1 1/2 C.   BUTTERMILK
1. Combine in a blender and process to liquefy.

HONEY OR BANANA AS NEEDED
2. Taste soup and sweeten with honey or banana if needed. Remember that this is not a dessert and should not be super sweet.

FRESH MINT AND/OR PIECES OF FRUIT
3. Serve in pretty glass bowls or sherbets garnished with mint and/or decorative slices of fruit or whole berries.

NOTE: This soup was developed to be used as a refreshing first course in the summer, but it also makes a great afternoon pick up. Serve it to your children and tell them it's a milk shake.

SHEILA'S FITNESS TIP: Walking does improve aerobic fitness. It has been found that even low intensity exercise reduces the risk of heart disease and cancer. Fifteen to seventeen minutes per mile is a good pace.

CARB 7 GM (65%)   PROTEIN 2 GM (21%)   FAT 1 GM (14%)   SODIUM 65 MG

GAZPACHO

MAKES 6 SERVINGS   20 CALORIES PER SERVING

2 T.   RED WINE VINEGAR
2 C.   TOMATO JUICE, UNSALTED
        1. Measure and place in a large pitcher.

1/4 C.   PARSLEY, FRESH
1/4 C.   SCALLIONS, CHOPPED
        2. With your food processor running, drop in the parsley and then the scallions to mince.
        3. Add the mixture to the tomato juice and mix well.

1/2 C.   FRESH TOMATO, CHOPPED
1/4 C.   GREEN BELL PEPPER, CHOPPED
1/2 C.   CUCUMBER, CHOPPED
        4. Hand chop, add to tomato juice and chill for at least an hour.

6   PARSLEY SPRIGS
1   LEMON, SLICED THIN
        5. Serve the Gazpacho in chilled bowls, topped with a slice of lemon and a sprig of parsley.

NOTE: This light and refreshing soup can become the star of your meal if you serve the chopped vegetables in bowls and let your guests help themselves. For a special occasion, try adding croutons and a bit of chopped avocado.

SHEILA'S FITNESS TIP: RACEWALK FOR FITNESS . . . Racewalking is a true calorie burner! It uses from 700 to 750 calories per hour, about 150 calories more per mile than jogging, and there's none of the bumping and bouncing that one experiences with jogging.

CARB 6 GM (81%)   PROTEIN 1 GM (15%)   FAT TRACE (4%)   SODIUM 35 MG

HEARTY BEAN SOUP

MAKES 12 SERVINGS   **250 CALORIES PER SERVING**

1	C.	LENTILS	1	C.	BLACK EYED PEAS
1	C.	YELLOW SPLIT PEAS	1	C.	KIDNEY BEANS
1	C.	GREEN SPLIT PEAS	1	C.	PINTO BEANS
1	C.	BABY LIMA BEANS	4	QT.	WATER
1	C.	NAVY BEANS			

1. Rinse the above and discard any debris.
2. Combine with water in a large soup kettle and soak overnight.

4	QT.	WATER	2	C.	ONION, CHOPPED
1		BAY LEAF			
1/4	C.	BERNARD JENSEN'S BROTH POWDER			

3. In the morning, drain the beans and add fresh water with the above ingredients.
4. Bring to a simmer, cover kettle and cook until beans are tender and peas are falling apart to thicken soup, 2 to 3 hours.

1	C.	PARSLEY, MINCED	1	C.	SCALLIONS, CHOPPED FINE

5. Mix in right before serving.

1/2	C.	PARMESAN CHEESE, GRATED

6. Serve soup in heated bowls with a sprinkle of cheese.

NOTE: This high protein, low fat and very delicious soup is a fine dish to have stored in your freezer for some non-cooking meals.

SHEILA'S FITNESS TIP: Remember to balance your exercise program with good nutrition. Make sure you are doing weight-bearing activities such as walking, along with taking the proper amount of calcium. This helps prevent osteoporosis.

CARB 36 GM (63%)   PROTEIN 16 GM (29%)   FAT 2 GM (8%)   SODIUM 92 MG

MINESTRONE

MAKES 6 SERVINGS   **120 CALORIES PER SERVING**

1	C.	TOMATO PASTE
3	C.	WATER
1/4	C.	BERNARD JENSEN'S BROTH POWDER
1/2	C.	ONION, MINCED
1	TSP.	GARLIC, FRESH PRESSED
1/2	TSP.	BASIL
1/2	TSP.	OREGANO
1	TSP.	CHILI POWDER (OPTIONAL, BUT GOOD)

1. Combine in soup kettle and bring to a simmer.

1	C.	POTATO, DICED
3	C.	MIXED FRESH VEGIES (ZUCCHINI, EGGPLANT, PEPPERS, CARROTS, MUSHROOMS, ETC.)
1/2	C.	PASTA TWISTS, BOWS OR SHELLS
1/2	C.	KIDNEY BEANS, COOKED

2. Add to kettle and simmer until tender.

1/2	C.	PARMESAN CHEESE, GRATED

3. Serve the soup in heated bowls topped with a sprinkle of cheese.

NOTE: Save your left over pasta and beans for this great main dish soup. It is a super "clean out the refrigerator" dish and makes a fine meal with a crunchy green salad and some wonderful whole grain bread.

SHEILA'S FITNESS TIP: Tackle temporary gain as it occurs. Weigh yourself once every two weeks and if there's more than a five pound difference, energize your metabolism with exercise. I recommend 40 minutes of brisk exercise, such as walking, dancing or a sport, 4 times a week.

CARB 22 GM (70%)   PROTEIN 6 GM (18%)   FAT 1 GM (12%)   SODIUM 100 MG

ONION SOUP PARMESAN

MAKES 6 HALF CUP SERVINGS   **20 CALORIES PER SERVING**

1/2	T.	WHITE WINE
1/2	T.	BUTTER BUDS
1	C.	ONION, CHOPPED

1. Combine wine and Butter Buds in a pan and heat; add onion and saute.

1/2	T.	LOW SODIUM SOY SAUCE
1/2	T.	ONION POWDER
3	C.	SOUP STOCK

2. Add to soup pot, bring to a simmer and cook for 30 minutes.

| 3 | T. | PARMESAN CHEESE, GRATED |
| 2 | T. | FRESH CHIVES, MINCED |

3. Serve the soup in heated bowls topped with 1/2 of a tablespoon of cheese and a sprinkle of chives

NOTE: This easy and delicious soup is an excellent first course or accompaniment to a hearty sandwich. If you can grate your own Parmesan cheese, it will have better flavor and a more elegant appearance.

SHEILA'S FITNESS TIP: For those who love statistics, it's been found that 53 percent of couples who lived with one another for over five years, shared the same exercise patterns. So, if you're just entering a new relationship, find an activity to share ... you'll encourage each other in all areas of your lives toward a more productive and zestful future ... together.

CARB 2 GM (45%)   PROTEIN 1 GM (25%)   FAT TRACE (30%)   SODIUM 40 MG

POTASSIUM BROTH

1/2	C.	POTATO, RED OR WHITE ROSE, DICED
2 1/2	C.	MIXED FRESH VEGIES (CARROT, SUMMER SQUASH, CELERY, PEAS, BROCCOLI, SPINACH, CHARD, ETC.)
2 1/2	C.	WATER

1. Combine and cook until vegies are tender.

2. Cool and puree in blender. (The soup should be very smooth. If there are strings from celery or any other lumps or bumps, strain the soup.)

3. Reheat in microwave or sauce pan, taste and add BERNARD JENSEN'S broth powder or herb seasoning, as needed.

TO MICROWAVE: Place washed vegies and potato in a plastic bag and microwave 4 minutes. Turn and microwave for 2 more minutes. Puree in blender with the water.

NOTE: This is an amazingly satisfying pick-up. We serve it at The Oaks/Palms as a mid-morning snack and it keeps everyone going very nicely. Try freezing it in little cups and use it when you feel like you could eat the whole refrigerator.

SHEILA'S FITNESS TIP: To strengthen the low back and abdominals, lie on your back with knees bent. Press the small of your back into the floor, pull your abdominals toward your backbone, contract your buttocks and hold for a count of eight. Repeat four more times.

CARB 3 GM (79%)   PROTEIN 1 GM (17%)   FAT TRACE (4%)   SODIUM 12 MG

SPLIT PEA SOUP

MAKES 10 SERVINGS   **90 CALORIES PER SERVING**

1 1/2	C.	GREEN SPLIT PEAS
2	QT.	BOILING WATER
1	C.	CELERY, CHOPPED
1	C.	CARROT, CHOPPED
1/2	C.	ONION, CHOPPED
1/4	TSP.	THYME, DRIED AND GROUND
2		BAY LEAVES
1/8	TSP.	CAYENNE

1. Combine in a kettle and return to a boil.
2. Reduce to a simmer and cook for 1 hour or until the split peas are tender.
3. Cool the soup and then puree.
4. Season to taste with BERNARD JENSEN'S BROTH POWDER, reheat and serve in heated soup bowls.

NOTE: This is one of our favorite main dish soups. It is satisfying and digestible. Paired with a salad filled pita, it becomes a meal that is faster than the fastest fast food with almost no dishes to wash.

SHEILA'S FITNESS TIP: To strengthen shoulders for a powerful swing in squash, tennis, racquetball or golf, try this: Use a light weight and lift with straightened arms to shoulder level. Keep thumbs down and arms in front of you. Lower arms and repeat ten times.

CARB 18 GM (73%)   PROTEIN 6 GM (23%)   FAT TRACE (4%)   SODIUM 15 MG

TOMATO CABBAGE SOUP

MAKES 6 SERVINGS   **40 CALORIES PER SERVING**

5	C.	TOMATO JUICE, UNSALTED

1. Place in sauce pan and bring to a simmer.

1	C.	CABBAGE, CHOPPED COARSELY
1/2	C.	ONION, MINCED
1/2	C.	CELERY, SLICED
1/4	TSP.	BASIL
1		BAY LEAF
1	TSP.	GARLIC, PRESSED
1	TSP.	RED WINE VINEGAR

2. Add to tomato juice and simmer for 1 hour.

2	T.	BERNARD JENSEN'S BROTH POWDER
2	T.	CHIVES, CHOPPED

3. Season with broth powder and serve in heated bowls topped with a sprinkle of chives.

NOTE: This simple soup really hits the spot on a cold day. Add a salad or sandwich and luncheon is served. Isn't it great to discover that a soup with only a trace of fat can be so satisfying?

SHEILA'S FITNESS TIP: It takes the body 20 minutes to signal the brain that you've eaten enough. Take smaller bites and concentrate on chewing longer.

CARB 10 GM (82%)   **PROTEIN 2 GM (15%)**   **FAT TRACE (3%)**   **SODIUM 70 MG**

TURKEY SOUP

MAKES 12 SERVINGS   **100 CALORIES PER SERVING**

3	QT.	WATER
1		TURKEY CARCASS (PULL OFF MEAT AND RESERVE)
2		BAY LEAVES

1. Combine in a large kettle and simmer for 3-4 hours.
2. Cool and refrigerate.
3. Lift off the hardened fat and remove bones, skin and bay leaves.

2	C.	CELERY, SLICED

4. Add to kettle and simmer for 15 minutes.

2	T.	ARROWROOT

5. Combine and stir into soup, heating and stirring to thicken the broth slightly.

3	C.	TURKEY MEAT RESERVED FROM CARCASS (OR MORE)
2	C.	FRESH MUSHROOMS, SLICED

6. Add to soup and simmer for 10 minutes more.

1/2	C.	FRESH PARSLEY

7. Serve in heated bowls and garnish soup with fresh snipped parsley.

NOTE: I usually add some cooked barley, rice or noodles with the turkey. If I happen to have any left over mashed potatoes, I thicken the broth with potato instead of arrowroot. I use turkey soup to clean out my refrigerator after Thanksgiving the way I use Minestrone at other times. In other words, put in anything you want. You may create a new recipe.

SHEILA'S FITNESS TIP: Dark turkey meat is higher in fat and cholesterol than white meat so leave the drum sticks for the children and enjoy the tender breast meat...with some delicious CRANBERRY GLAZE. (DRESSINGS, DIPS AND SPREADS)

CARB 6 GM (25%)   PROTEIN 12 GM (53%)   FAT 2 GM (22%)   SODIUM 52 MG

WINTER SQUASH SOUP

MAKES 6 HALF CUP SERVINGS   **25 CALORIES PER SERVING**

1 1/2 C. **WINTER SQUASH, CHOPPED IN SMALL PIECES**
            1. Peel, chop, measure and place in sauce pan.

1/4 C. **ONION, CHOPPED**
1/4 C. **BELL PEPPER, CHOPPED (USE YELLOW IF AVAILABLE)**
1 1/2 C. **CHICKEN OR VEGETABLE STOCK**
            2. Add to sauce pan, bring stock to a boil and cook until the vegetables are tender.
            3. Cool, place in blender and process smooth.

1/2 TSP. **CINNAMON**   1/2 TSP   **NUTMEG**
1/2 TSP. **CUMIN**   1/2 TSP. **CORIANDER**
1/4 TSP. **CURRY OR GARAM MASALA**
1 T. **BERNARD JENSEN'S BROTH POWDER**
            4. Add to blender contents, process to mix and return soup to sauce pan to heat.

2 T. **NONFAT YOGURT**   2 TSP. **CHIVES, MINCED**
            5. Serve the soup in heated bowls topped with a teaspoon of yogurt and a sprinkle of chives.

NOTE: If you have an abundance of squash, double or triple this recipe and freeze some. Winter squash is one of the best sources of immune system building Beta Carotene so serve this soup often. I sometimes use carrot instead of some or all of the squash. It produces a somewhat sweeter soup. If you have purchased or made some Garam Masala, it is a very delicious seasoning...milder and sweeter than most curry mixtures.

SHEILA'S FITNESS TIP: To stay motivated, think of movements as a positive habit. Make one of your habits taking stairs rather than elevators.

CARB 5 GM (76%)   **PROTEIN 1 GM (12%)**   **FAT TRACE (11%)**   **SODIUM 5 MG**

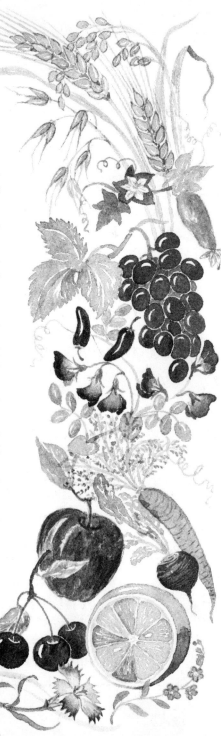

SCRUMPTIOUS SALADS

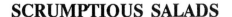

Many people believe that the word salad means low calorie. Since most salad dressings are over 90% fat nothing could be farther from the truth . . . Except for the salads in this book.

Since we need green leafy vegetables every day, a tossed green salad is a most delightful way to please palate as well as dietary needs. Make sure your greens are dry and chilled, then toss with your favorite dressing and serve immediately. The Italian Dressing and Raspberry Vinaigrette in DRESSINGS, DIPS AND SPREADS are especially good on mixed greens.

When the weather turns warm, a main dish salad is an easy and healthy alternative to cooking. Put one together early in the day and enjoy knowing that your dinner is ready and waiting. The Crab Salad, Curried Lobster, Pasta Primavera, Sesame Chicken and Marinated Tuna Tofu are excellent when prepared ahead.

You will find a number of marinated vegetable salads that travel and wait well. Keep your favorites on hand for quick meals, pot lucks and picnics.

Many people fail to eat as many fresh fruits and vegetable as they need for optimum health. Make salads with the freshest ingredients you can find part of your ULTIMATE RECIPE FOR FITNESS.

ANTIPASTO SALAD

1/2 C.   TOMATO JUICE
  1 TSP. ARROWROOT
         1. Combine and cook and stir over low heat to thicken the juice.

  2 T.   OLIVES, SLICED   1 T.   BASIL, FRESH SNIPPED
1/4 C.   RED WINE VINEGAR   2 T.   SCALLIONS OR CHIVES, MINCED
1/4 C.   BALSAMIC VINEGAR   1 T.   PARSLEY, MINCED
1/2 TSP. OREGANO, FRESH SNIPPED
         2. Mix with thickened tomato juice and set aside.

  2 C.   BELL PEPPERS, CUT IN 1 INCH CUBES, MIXED COLORS IF POSSIBLE
  1 C.   CARROTS, CUT ON A DIAGONAL
  1 C.   CAULIFLOWER, BROKEN INTO FLOWERETTES
         3. Combine and steam for 3 minutes.
         4. Toss hot vegetables with dressing.

 12   MED. MUSHROOMS, CLEANED AND SCORED ON TOP
  8 OZ. CAN OF ARTICHOKE HEARTS, HALVED
         5. Add to vegetable mixture and marinate for at least two hours.

  1 HD. SALAD BOWL LETTUCE
         6. Line bowl or individual plates with large leaves and fill with small leaves.
         7. Arrange Antipasto on top of lettuce in an attractive manner.

NOTE: This is a light and lovely beginning to an Italian dinner.

SHEILA'S FITNESS TIP: To help control your percentage of body fat (most people call it 'weight'), combine the use of these recipes with a vigorous 20 minute walk after each meal.

CARB 8 GM (70%)   PROTEIN 2 GM (16%)   FAT 1 GM (14%)   SODIUM 72 MG

APPLE CABBAGE SLAW VERONICA

MAKES 6 SERVINGS   **35 CALORIES PER SERVING**

1/2	C.	NONFAT YOGURT
1/2	TSP.	LEMON ZEST (FRESH GRATED LEMON PEEL)
1/2	TSP.	LEMON JUICE
1/2	TSP.	HONEY

1. Combine and mix well for dressing.

1 1/2	C.	CABBAGE, GRATED
1/2	C.	ORANGE, SECTIONED AND SLICED
1/2	C.	GRAPES, HALVED
1/4	C.	CELERY, SLICED THIN
1/2	C.	RED APPLE, DICED

2. Combine and toss with dressing right before serving.

6	LETTUCE LEAVES

3. Scoop salad into a lettuce leaf and serve.

NOTE: If you are not going to serve this right away, cover and chill the dressing and salad separately. This salad travels well so you might want to take it to a pot luck, a picnic or even to work.

SHEILA'S FITNESS TIP: Know that in your quest to change your habits, lose weight and exercise more, occasionally, you are going to fall off of the wagon. If you realize this in the beginning, you will forgive yourself, and get back on again.... You're human ... you're allowed mistakes.

CARB 8 GM (80%)   **PROTEIN 2 GM (16%)**   **FAT TRACE (4%)**   **SODIUM 23 MG**

BEET & ONION SALAD, MARINATED

MAKES 6 SERVINGS   **25 CALORIES PER SERVING**

2 C.   **COOKED BEETS, FRESH OR CANNED AND RINSED**
1. Slice thin and place in a bowl.

1 C.   **RED ONION**
2. Slice paper thin and add to beets.

1/4 C.   **CIDER VINEGAR**
2 T.   **LEMON JUICE, FRESH**
1 TSP.   **HONEY**
3. Combine, pour over beet mixture, cover and chill.
4. After about an hour, mix and toss so that marinade is well distributed.
5. Serve over lettuce as a salad.

NOTE: This may be served with a dollop of lowcal sour cream. It is also very nice served as a relish, side dish or even as a topping for an open faced Scandinavian type sandwich.

CARB 6 GM (87%)   **PROTEIN 1 GM (11%)**   **FAT TRACE (2%)**   **SODIUM 28 MG**

CALORIE CONSCIOUS COBB SALAD

MAKES 8 SERVINGS   **200 CALORIES PER SERVING**

1 LB. TOFU
1. Drain and press out as much water as possible.
2. Slice in thin strips to resemble slices of bacon and place in a shallow pan.

1/2 C. LOW SODIUM SOY SAUCE
1 1/3 T. BAKON YEAST (AVAILABLE IN HEALTH FOOD STORES)
3. Combine and sprinkle over tofu.
4. Marinate for one hour and place under broiler until tofu browns. Set aside to cool and then crumble to resemble bacon bits.

8   LEAVES OF SALAD BOWL LETTUCE   **1/2 C. CRABMEAT, SHREDDED**
8 C. ICEBERG LETTUCE, CHOPPED   **4 OZ. MOZZARELLA, GRATED**
2 C. TOMATO, DICED
2 OZ. BLUE CHEESE, CRUMBLED AND MIXED WITH THE MOZZARELLA
1 C. SCALLIONS, CHOPPED

5. To prepare individual salads, mound chopped lettuce on large leaves on salad plates.
6. Arrange the other ingredients in strips over the lettuce so that the chopped lettuce is almost hidden.
7. Serve with AVOCADO SALAD DRESSING (DRESSINGS, DIPS & SPREADS).

NOTE: There are many options available to you in converting this salad to include your favorite ingredients. This is the version we serve at The Oaks and it is greatly enjoyed by our guests.

SHEILA'S FITNESS TIP: Dining out? Pizza get's 36% of it's calories from fat, however the sandwich that the diet-conscious person often chooses (a tuna sandwich) gets 46% of it's calories from fat-mostly because of the mayonnaise.

CARB 7 GM (21%)   PROTEIN 17 GM (47%)   FAT 5 GM (33%)   SODIUM 500 MG

CARROT DATE SALAD WITH WALNUTS

MAKES 1 MAIN DISH SALAD   **295 CALORIES PER SERVING**

2	C.	**CARROT, GRATED**
5		**DATES, CHOPPED OR SLICED**

1. Grate carrots into bowl and slice dates over carrots.

2	T.	**WALNUTS**

2. Chop walnuts and toast under broiler to brown.
3. Sprinkle walnuts over the salad right before serving.

NOTE: This salad is a personal favorite of mine and I purchased a Salad Shooter just to make it easy to have a quick carrot salad anytime I want. It is best eaten immediately after you make it. Since the protein is low, I usually have a glass of skim milk with it.

SHEILA'S FITNESS TIP: Feeling a little tension in the neck? Say "yes" 10 times, "no" 10 times — repeat again.

CARB 54 GM (67%)   **PROTEIN 5 GM (6%)**   **FAT 9 GM (26%)**   **SODIUM 80 MG**

CRAB SALAD

MAKES 10 SERVINGS   **100 CALORIES PER SERVING**

1	QT.	LOWFAT COTTAGE CHEESE (1%)
1	C.	CRAB MEAT, (IMITATION CRAB WORKS WELL)
2	T.	LOWCAL MAYONNAISE, (FROM THIS BOOK OR COMMERCIAL)
1/4	C.	PARSLEY, CHOPPED
2	T.	SCALLIONS, MINCED

1. Combine all ingredients and mix well.
2. Cover and chill.
3. Serve stuffed into an artichoke or tomato set on a bed of lettuce ... or serve on a bed of lettuce and garnish with tomato wedges and artichoke hearts ... or stuff into a Pita Bread with lettuce and tomato.

NOTE: The possibilities for this delicious mixture are endless. It takes about 5 minutes to prepare and everyone likes it. It is my personal favorite for those days when I don't feel like cooking or eating out.

SHEILA'S FITNESS TIP: Some people falsely believe that they lose body weight after a stay in the sauna, steam room or hot tub. Not so! All that is lost is water from the body cells and as soon as we take a drink of water those cells replenish the water loss, much like a dry sponge instantly fills with liquid.

CARB 4 GM (16%)   PROTEIN 15 GM (61%)   FAT 2 GM (23%)   SODIUM 511 MG

CURRIED LOBSTER IN PAPAYA SALAD

MAKES 6 SERVINGS   **165 CALORIES PER SERVING**

3		PAPAYA, RIPE , HALVED AND SEEDED
1		LEMON OR LIME

1. Sprinkle the papaya with lemon or lime juice and chill.

1	LB.	LOBSTER CHUNKS (OR USE HALF WHITE FISH AND HALF LOBSTER)
1/4	C.	SCALLIONS, MINCED
2	T.	LEMON JUICE, FRESH

2. Combine and fill papaya shells with mixture.

1/2	TSP.	CANOLA OIL
1	T.	SCALLIONS, MINCED
1	T.	CURRY POWDER

3. Heat oil and cook onion and curry powder to a paste.

1/2		BANANA (VERY RIPE)

4. Blend in blender until smooth.

1/2	C.	NONFAT YOGURT

5. Add to banana with curry paste and process smooth.
6. Chill, place fruit and lobster mixture on lettuce leaves and serve with dressing spooned over the lobster.

NOTE: Sometimes if your papayas are not quite ripe, you can complete the ripening in your Microwave. Simply cover or place in a plastic bag after sprinkling on the lime or lemon juice. Microwave for about a minute, chill and proceed.

> SHEILA'S FITNESS TIP: It's important to wear the right shoe for the right sport. Do not attempt to wear tennis shoes for running or running shoes for tennis.

CARB 17 GM (40%)   **PROTEIN 22 GM (53%)**   **FAT 1 GM (8%)**   **SODIUM 112 MG**

CURRIED TUNA SALAD

MAKES 2 SERVINGS   195 CALORIES PER SERVING

1	6 OZ. CAN WATER PACKED TUNA
1	MED. PIPPIN OR GRANNY SMITH APPLE, DICED 1/4 INCH
4	WATER CHESTNUTS, DICED 1/4 INCH
2	SCALLIONS, CHOPPED FINE

1. Combine in a large bowl, mixing lightly to leave some large pieces of tuna.

1/4	C.	LOWCAL MAYONNAISE
1/2	TSP.	CURRY POWDER

2. Combine and mix lightly with tuna mixture.

2   LARGE LETTUCE LEAVES

3. Serve on lettuce leaves with any of the following optional ingredients:

RAISINS
CHUTNEY OR TRY THE PINEAPPLE MARMALADE (see DRESSINGS, DIPS
AND SPREADS)
NONFAT YOGURT

NOTE: At The Oaks, we serve this with a half a Pita and some of the condiments listed above. It has been a huge success. It would also be wonderful accompanied by a fresh fruit salad. If you are a lover of curry, you may want to increase the amount of curry powder. The rather modest amount used here is meant to please the average palate.

SHEILA'S FITNESS TIP: Here is a fitness move to trim your bottom. Contract all the muscles in your rear. Standing, bend your knees slightly and hold the muscles in your rear tight for a slow count of 10. Release and repeat 5 more times.

CARB 23 GM (40%)   PROTEIN 27 GM (49%)   FAT 3 GM (11%)   SODIUM 155 MG

FRESH MUSHROOM SALAD

MAKES 6 SERVINGS   **20 CALORIES PER SERVING**

1/2	T.	ARROWROOT
1/2	C.	WATER

1. Whisk together in a small sauce pan, heat and stir to thicken.

TO MICROWAVE: Whisk together in a glass measuring cup and microwave one minute to thicken. Whisk again and microwave for another half minute if needed.

1	TSP.	CANOLA OIL
6	T.	WHITE WINE VINEGAR
1 1/2	T.	PARMESAN CHEESE, GRATED
1	TSP.	FRESH GARLIC, PRESSED
2	T.	FRESH PARSLEY, MINCED
2	T.	SCALLIONS, MINCED
2	TSP.	BAKON YEAST (AVAILABLE IN HEALTH FOOD STORES)

2. Whisk into the thickened water and set aside.

2	C.	FRESH MUSHROOMS, CLEANED

3. Slice across and marinate in the dressing for at least an hour.

12		BIBB LETTUCE LEAVES OR AN EQUAL AMOUNT OF FRESH SPINACH

4. Arrange on individual salad plates and top with the marinated mushrooms.

NOTE: This is one of my favorite salads but it's not very colorful. Find a brightly colored garnish such as red bell pepper or cherry tomato and serve to your favorite guests. We usually serve this as the salad course at The Oaks for Thanksgiving dinner because it leaves a lot of calories to spend elsewhere.

SHEILA'S FITNESS TIP: Get serious about your body. Pamper it. Know that pain is an early warning that something is WRONG and NOT that you're supposed to work harder.

CARB 2 GM (29%)   PROTEIN 2 GM (28%)   FAT 1 GM (43%)   SODIUM 24 MG

HERBED RED POTATO SALAD

MAKES 6 SERVINGS   **80 CALORIES PER SERVING**

3 C. **RED POTATOES, SCRUBBED CLEAN...DO NOT PEEL**
1. Boil or steam until tender.
TO MICROWAVE: Wash, place in plastic bag and microwave until tender (18 to 20 minutes).

1/4 C. **RED ONION, MINCED AND SOAKED 1/2 HOUR IN ICE WATER**
1/4 C. **PARSLEY, MINCED**
2 T. **CHIVES, MINCED...GARLIC CHIVES IF AVAILABLE**
1 T. **FRESH DILL, MINCED OR 1 TSP. DRIED DILL**
2. Cut potatoes in bite sized pieces and place in bowl.
3. Toss with herbs and drained onion.

1 C. **LOWCAL SOUR CREAM (see DRESSINGS, DIPS AND SPREADS)**
1 T. **BALSAMIC VINEGAR**
1 TSP. **BERNARD JENSEN'S BROTH POWDER**
4. Combine for dressing and toss with potatoes.
5. Cover and chill.
6. Serve garnished with sprigs of fresh dill or parsley.

NOTE: This is a refreshing and light change from the usual old fashioned mayonnaise laden, sweet pickle filled salad that our grandmothers took to picnics. Feel free to add or subtract herbs but try to use fresh herbs.

SHEILA'S FITNESS TIP: Having trouble deciding what to eat when away from your own kitchen? Here's a good rule of thumb. Try to avoid the FOUR BAD WHITES; sugar, salt, flour and fat.

CARB 18 GM (87%)   **PROTEIN 2 GM (12%)**   **FAT TRACE (2%)**   **SODIUM 9 MG**

HIGH FIBER SALAD

1	C.	RED OR GREEN CABBAGE, CHOPPED
1		APPLE, CHOPPED
1	C.	CARROT, GRATED

1. Combine in a large salad bowl.

1		ORANGE, PEELED AND CHOPPED
1	OZ.	SUNFLOWER SEEDS
1/2	C.	SPROUTS (ALFALFA OR MIXED)

2. Arrange over cabbage mixture and eat promptly.

NOTE: This salad is one of the alternates always available for lunch and/or dinner at The Oaks and Palms. Guests might choose a CLEANSING DAY and order this for lunch and dinner which usually leaves them feeling light and lively. Try it the next time you feel heavy from over indulging. If you are dining alone and want a meal that is easily prepared in one bowl, this is it. Along with a lot of fiber, this salad has the added benefit of supplying 100% of the RDA for vitamins A and C as well as 92% of vitamin E. That makes this salad a super booster of the immune system.

SHEILA'S FITNESS TIP: When you feed your body properly, you'll have more quick and enduring energy. You'll want to put more muscle into a workout because you'll feel more energetic. When you're energetic, your muscles, including heart and lungs will get a far better workout and you'll become stronger . . . SO EAT RIGHT and DON'T DIET.

CARB 45 GM (71%)   PROTEIN 8 GM (11%)   FAT 5 GM (19%)   SODIUM 42 MG

MARINATED TUNA TOFU SALAD

MAKES 8 SERVINGS   215 CALORIES PER SERVING

1 LB. FIRM TOFU
1. Drain and press out water. Place several layers of paper towels under and over the tofu and top with a weight.

2 T.	**DRY SHERRY**	**1/2 TSP. GARLIC, PRESSED**
2 T.	**WATER**	**1/16 TSP. ANISE, GROUND**
1 TSP.	**HONEY**	**1/16 TSP. BLACK PEPPER**
2 T.	**SOY SAUCE, LOW SODIUM**	**1/2 TSP. SESAME OIL**
2 T.	**CIDER VINEGAR**	

2. Combine and mix well for marinade.
3. Cut tofu into half inch pieces, place in a shallow pan and pour marinade over the tofu. Marinate for several hours or overnight.

2 CANS WATER PACKED TUNA   **1/3 C. SCALLIONS, MINCED**
(6 TO 7 OZ. SIZE)   **1/4 C. LOWCAL MAYONNAISE**
2/3 C. CELERY, SLICED THIN ON A DIAGONAL
5. Combine and mix gently to keep the tuna in bite sized pieces.
6. Add the tofu with the marinade and mix gently.

8 PURPLE CABBAGE LEAVES   **2 C. SHREDDED CABBAGE**
3 T. WALNUTS, CHOPPED AND TOASTED
7. Fill cabbage leaves with shredded cabbage and top with the tuna tofu mixture and add walnuts.

NOTE: At The Oaks, we serve this with half of a Mini Whole Wheat Pita.

SHEILA'S FITNESS TIP: Monitor your workout shoes. If shoes are wearing down one section of the sole, talk to a Podiatrist.

CARB 18 GM (33%)   PROTEIN 22 GM (40%)   FAT 7 GM (27%)   SODIUM 77 MG

MEXICAN ORANGE ONION SALAD

MAKES 8 SERVINGS   **50 CALORIES PER SERVING**

1	TSP.	CANOLA OIL	1/3	TSP.	CUMIN
2/3	TSP.	ONION POWDER	1/3	TSP.	GARLIC POWDER
2/3	TSP.	CHILI POWDER	1/3	TSP.	OREGANO

1. Drop oil in sauce pan, heat and add seasonings to heat through.

1/3	C.	WHITE VINEGAR	1	TSP.	LEMON JUICE
1/2	TSP.	HONEY	1/2	C.	WATER

2. Add to pan and heat to just below boiling.

1	TSP.	ARROWROOT	2	T.	ORANGE JUICE

3. Combine and whisk smooth.
4. Add to sauce pan, heat and stir to thicken dressing.
5. Chill dressing.

4 C. BIBB OR BRONZE LEAF LETTUCE, TORN INTO BITE SIZED PIECES
2 C. ORANGE SLICES
1 C. PURPLE ONION, SLICED VERY THIN AND SOAKED IN ICE WATER 1 HOUR

6. Toss with dressing just before serving.

NOTE: We get requests for the dressing when we serve this salad at the Spas. The combination of orange and purple onion seems just right with Mexican food.

SHEILA'S FITNESS TIP: Indoor exercise bicycles provide a good workout for someone recovering from an illness, pregnancy or surgery. When selecting a bike, try out different models and choose one that has variable tension so that you can make the ride more difficult as you become stronger. Select a bike with a comfortable seat as well. After the first five miles, you'll be glad you did.

CARB 11 GM (78%)   PROTEIN 1 GM (9%)   FAT 1 GM (13%)   SODIUM 5 MG

ORANGE ZUCCHINI SALAD

MAKES 6 SERVINGS   **50 CALORIES PER SERVING**

1/4 C.	WHITE VINEGAR	
1 TSP.	HONEY	
1 TSP.	CANOLA OIL	
3 1/2 OZ.	WATER	
1/8 TSP.	BLACK PEPPER	

1/2 TSP.	ONION POWDER
1/2 TSP.	CUMIN
1/4 TSP.	GARLIC POWDER
1/8 TSP.	OREGANO
1 TSP.	ARROWROOT

1. Combine in a sauce pan, heat and stir to thicken.
TO MICROWAVE: Combine in a glass bowl or measuring cup and microwave for 2-3 minutes. Remove and whisk.

1 T.   ORANGE JUICE
1 TSP.   LEMON JUICE

2. Add to dressing and chill.

2 C.   ORANGE, SLICED THIN
1 C.   PURPLE ONION, SLICED VERY THIN
2 C.   ZUCCHINI, SLICED THIN

3. Combine in a flat bottom bowl, pour dressing over all and marinate for at least an hour.

6   LARGE LETTUCE CUPS

4. Spoon into lettuce cups right before serving.

NOTE: This is an outstanding salad. However, it's success is dependent upon very fresh zucchini and flavorful oranges.

SHEILA'S FITNESS TIP: Drink plenty of water. Drink before, during and after exercise. Remember, thirst is a learned response. You can override it and become dehydrated.

CARB 12 GM (79%)   **PROTEIN 1 GM (10%)**   **FAT 1 GM (12%)**   **SODIUM 3 MG**

ORIENTAL CUCUMBER SALAD

MAKES 8 SERVINGS   **10 CALORIES PER SERVING**

3   **CUCUMBERS (SCRUB TO REMOVE ANY WAX)**
           1. Halve and remove seeds.
           2. Slice very thin, cutting on a diagonal and place in a bowl.

2 T.   **RICE VINEGAR**
1/3 TSP. **PEPPER, FRESH GROUND**
1/2 TSP. **SESAME OIL**
           3. Combine, mix well and toss with cucumber slices.
           4. Cover and chill for at least an hour.

8   **BAK CHOY OR CHINESE CABBAGE LEAVES**
           5. Serve the cucumbers on the leaves on chilled salad plates.

NOTE: This lightest of salads is a most refreshing way to begin an Oriental or Middle Eastern meal.

SHEILA'S FITNESS TIP: If you exercise outdoors, use a sunscreen to prevent premature aging or abnormal cell formation. However, don't stay inside the gym or in your living room during every session because the sun is actually wonderful. According to the results of research in Germany, sunshine may be related to the production of painkilling hormones known as endorphins. The body increases production of these when you exercise in the sun. In addition, sunlight kills some bacteria and it's been used as effective treatment for psoriasis.

CARB 2 GM (60%)   PROTEIN 1/4 GM (60%)   FAT 1/3 GM (29%)   SODIUM 5 MG

ORIENTAL RICE SALAD

MAKES 8 SERVINGS   **105 CALORIES PER SERVING**

2	C.	**BROWN RICE, COOKED**
1	C.	**MUSHROOMS, SLICED**
1	C.	**SNOW PEAS OR EDIBLE PEA PODS**
1	C.	**CELERY, SLICED THIN ON A DIAGONAL**
1/2	C.	**RED BELL PEPPER, SLIVERED**
1/2	C.	**SCALLIONS, MINCED**

1. Combine and toss lightly

1	T.	**SESAME OIL**
1/4	C.	**RICE VINEGAR**
2	T.	**LOW SODIUM SOY SAUCE**

2. Combine and mix well.
3. Toss dressing with rice mixture and chill.

1/4	C.	**ALMONDS, TOASTED AND SLIVERED**

NOTE: This is an excellent salad to have on the day following a Chinese dinner. Simply combine your left over rice with your left over stir fried vegies, add a few raw scallions and celery bits for crunch, mix the dressing and toss. If you do this while you are cleaning up from the Chinese meal you won't have to cook the next night. Add any chicken, shrimp or lobster that you have left also.

SHEILA'S FITNESS TIP: When buying a workout video, read the label and make sure the one you choose is right for your present fitness level. Before you begin, dress for the occasion, especially shoe-wise, and open windows for good air circulation or turn on a fan.

CARB 15 MG (56%)   **PROTEIN 3 GM (10%)**   **FAT 4 GM (34%)**   **SODIUM 20 MG**

PASTA PRIMAVERA SALAD WITH CHEESE

MAKES 6 SERVINGS   **220 CALORIES PER SERVING**

1/2 LB. PASTA TWISTS
1. Cook in boiling water according to directions on the package.
2. Transfer to a colander and rinse under cold running water.

1/4 C. ITALIAN DRESSING (see DRESSINGS, DIPS AND SPREADS)
3. Toss cooked pasta with dressing in salad bowl.

1/2 C. CARROTS, GRATED
1/2 C. RED BELL PEPPER, SLICED IN 1/4 INCH PIECES
1/2 C. ARTICHOKE HEARTS, COOKED AND QUARTERED
3 OZ. LIFETIME CHEDDAR CHEESE, CUBED IN 1/4 INCH PIECES
3 OZ. LIFETIME SWISS CHEESE, CUBED IN 1/4 INCH PIECES
1/4 C. DRIED TOMATOES, STEAMED TO SOFTEN AND CUT INTO 1/4 INCH PIECES
4. Toss with warm pasta and dressing.
5. Cover and chill for at least two hours. Overnight is better.

2 C. CHERRY TOMATOES, HALVED
12 LETTUCE LEAVES
2 T. PARMESAN CHEESE, GRATED
6. Serve the salad on lettuce leaves and top with a sprinkle of cheese. Moisten with more dressing if needed. Garnish with cherry tomatoes.

NOTE: Feel free to use any Italian Dressing you have on hand for this. You can also add or subtract ingredients. This salad is a good place to use leftovers.

SHEILA'S FITNESS TIP: Hold in your stomach for health. The simple act of contracting the abdominal muscles will build a support system for your entire torso and back.

CARB 31 GM (53%)   PROTEIN 15 GM (25%)   FAT 6 GM (22%)   SODIUM 101 MG

SAMBALS (INDIAN SALAD)

MAKES 12 SERVINGS   30 CALORIES PER SERVING

1	C.	CUCUMBER

1. Halve, remove seeds and slice. Place in a salad bowl.

2	C.	TOMATO CHUNKS
1	C.	GREEN BEANS, MINCED
1	C.	BELL PEPPERS, CUBED
1	C.	GREEN PEAS

2. Toss with cucumber.

1	C.	RED ONION. SLICED THIN

3. Place in a small bowl and cover with ice water.

2	T.	LEMON JUICE
2	T.	RICE VINEGAR
1	TSP.	PEPPER, FRESH GROUND
1	TSP.	BERNARD JENSEN'S BROTH POWDER

4. Mix together for marinade or dressing.

1/4	C.	PARSLEY, MINCED

5. Drain onion and toss with the rest of the Sambals along with the parsley.
6. Toss with dressing and cover and chill.
7. Serve with Indian food.

NOTE: Use your imagination and taste buds to make up your own Sambals.

SHEILA'S FITNESS TIP: Attach a Fitness Habit to another habit. After you wash your face in the morning, do 20 push-aways at your bathroom counter. Use wasted moments to tone the body.

CARB 7 GM (80%)   PROTEIN 1 GM (16%)   FAT TRACE (4%)   SODIUM 15 MG

SEAFOOD PASTA SALAD

MAKES 6 SERVINGS   130 CALORIES PER SERVING

2	C.	PASTA TWISTS OR SEA SHELLS, COOKED
2	C.	SEAFOOD, COOKED (SALMON, SNAPPER, SOLE, SHRIMP, ETC.)
2	C.	CELERY, SLICED THIN ON A DIAGONAL
1/4	C.	SCALLIONS, MINCED
2	T.	PARSLEY, MINCED
1/2	C.	LEMON MAYONNAISE (see DRESSINGS, DIPS AND SPREADS)

1. Toss together and chill.
2. Serve on lettuce leaves or a bed of mixed greens.

NOTE: This recipe was designed to use leftover cooked seafood. However it would work equally well with canned or frozen seafood. If you cook some extra snapper or salmon the next time you have fish for dinner, you can prepare dinner for two nights at the same time. Pick up a little cooked bay shrimp and/or crab to add to your salad and you'll have a feast all ready to eat when you get home. If you don't like making your own mayonnaise, buy the lowcal variety and thin it down with fresh lemon juice.

SHEILA'S FITNESS TIP: A sound WELLNESS PROGRAM does not have to consume your life. Three 45 minute workouts per week, that include 20 minutes of aerobics in your target zone, tends to increase flexibility and strengthen the abdominals and upper torso. Now add 25 minutes of sports fitness; bicycling, volleyball, etc. Combined, these two types of exercise will do wonders for body and spirit.

CARB 12 GM (39%)   PROTEIN 17 GM (53%)   FAT 1 GM (9%)   SODIUM 88 MG

SESAME CHICKEN SALAD

MAKES 6 SERVINGS   **160 CALORIES PER SERVING**

1/4	C.	**LOW SODIUM SOY SAUCE**	1/4 C.	**DRY SHERRY**

1. Combine in a shallow dish for a marinade.

1 LB. CHICKEN TENDERS (BONELESS, SKINLESS CHICKEN PIECES)

2. Place in the shallow dish to marinate for 2 hours, turning once.

1 TSP. PEANUT OIL   **2 TSP. FRESH GARLIC, MINCED**
2 TSP. FRESH GINGER, MINCED

3. Saute garlic and ginger in hot oil, reserving 1 tsp. each for dressing.
4. Drain chicken.
5. Add chicken to pan and stir fry until opaque. Take care not to overcook.
6. Place chicken in a covered dish and chill.

3/4 C. WATER   **1/2 C. RICE VINEGAR**
1/4 C. HONEY   **1 TSP. RESERVED GINGER**
1 T. SESAME OIL   **1 TSP. RESERVED GARLIC**

7. Combine for dressing and chill.

1   HEAD LEAF LETTUCE, WASHED AND DRIED

8. Arrange on individual salad plates, using the large leaves as a nest.

18   CHINESE PEA PODS   **1/2 C. JICAMA, SLIVERED**
12 OZ. ENOKI MUSHROOMS   **2 T. TOASTED SESAME SEEDS**
1 1/2 C. BEAN SPROUTS

9. Arrange on lettuce, topping with chicken and sprinkling chicken with Sesame seeds. Garnish with the pea pods. Serve dressing on the side.

NOTE: This can also be placed in a salad bowl and tossed with the dressing right before serving.

CARB 14 GM (31%)   PROTEIN 16 GM (36%)   FAT 6 GM (33%)   SODIUM 247 MG

SPINACH SALAD

MAKES 6 SERVINGS   **65 CALORIES PER SERVING**

1/4	C.	WATER
2	T.	CANOLA OIL
1/4	C.	RICE VINEGAR (OR WHITE WINE VINEGAR)
2	T.	PARMESAN CHEESE, GRATED
1		CLOVE GARLIC, MINCED
1	T.	SMOKED YEAST (AVAILABLE IN HEALTH FOOD STORES)
1	T.	PARSLEY
1	T.	SCALLION

1. Combine in blender and process for dressing.
2. Refrigerate and chill.

6	C.	FRESH SPINACH, STEMS REMOVED AND TORN IN BITE SIZED PIECES
1 1/2	C.	MUSHROOMS, CLEANED AND SLICED
2		EGG WHITES, CHOPPED
2	T.	SCALLIONS, MINCED

3. Place spinach in a bowl and top with the other ingredients.
4. Toss with dressing and serve immediately.

NOTE: This can also be served as individual salads with 1 ounce of dressing on the side. The dressing is 45 calories per ounce so if you can get by with half the dressing, you will get rid of a lot of the fat calories. If you are serving this as a main dish salad, add some croutons, more egg and double the spinach.

SHEILA'S FITNESS TIP: Get a buddy to work out with. It will be easier to stay with your fitness goals if you're obligated to someone else.

CARB 4 GM (22%)   **PROTEIN 3 (18%)**   **FAT 5 GM (60%)**   **SODIUM 80 MG**

TOMATO, BASIL, MOZZARELLA SALAD

MAKES 6 SERVINGS   **45 CALORIES PER SERVING**

3	LG.	FRESH TOMATOES, SLICED 1/4 INCH THICK
3	OZ.	LIFETIME MOZZARELLA, SLICED VERY THIN
1/4	C.	FRESH BASIL LEAVES, SHREDDED
12		BIBB LETTUCE LEAVES

1. Arrange lettuce on a chilled salad plate; top with tomato, cheese and basil.
2. Serve as a first course or side dish.

NOTE: If fresh basil is not available, use 1 T. dried basil mixed with 3 T. chopped chives and/or parsley. Do not attempt this unless you have some good vine ripened tomatoes. We sometimes prepare this at The Oaks substituting a Mozzarella Creamy Cheese for the plain Mozzarella. See DRESSINGS, DIPS AND SPREADS for the recipe for CREAMY CHEESE.

SHEILA'S FITNESS TIP: Did you know that choosing an English muffin rather than a croissant will save you 95 calories and that corn flakes rather than granola can save over 200 calories?

CARB 9 GM (28%)   PROTEIN 6 GM (56%)   FAT 1 GM (15%)   SODIUM 165 MG

WINTER CARROUSEL

MAKES 6 SERVINGS   **25 CALORIES PER SERVING**

6 OZ.   CARROT
6 OZ.   RAW BEET
6 OZ.   RED CABBAGE
6 OZ.   JICAMA OR TURNIP
    1. Scrub vegetables and grate into 4 separate bowls. Take care to leave vegetables loose and not packed.

6   LARGE LETTUCE LEAVES
    2. Line 6 salad plates with lettuce and arrange an ounce of each grated vegetable carrousel style on the lettuce.

6 OZ.   RASPBERRY VINAIGRETTE (see DRESSINGS, DIPS & SPREADS)
    3. Serve with dressing on the side or toss each grated vegetable with dressing before serving. The salad is more visually appealing if the dressing is served on the side.

NOTE: Executive Chef David Del Nagro brought this lovely salad to The Oaks. We substituted the RASPBERRY VINAIGRETTE for a more traditional vinaigrette. The raspberry dressing has no oil so the calorie saving is substantial. Oil is fat and there is nothing more fattening than eating fat.

SHEILA'S FITNESS TIP: From now on, promise yourself that regardless of how expensive the meal is, you will leave 1/3 of everything on your plate or take home a doggie bag ... (for your DOGGIE?)

CARB 5 GM (88%)   PROTEIN 1 GM (10%)   FAT TRACE (2%)   SODIUM 35 MG

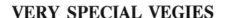

VERY SPECIAL VEGIES

This chapter includes many recipes for vegetarian entrees and since most of us eat too much meat and protein, we hope that you will find some favorites and serve them often.

The Fresh Mushroom Filets, Artichoke Chili Stuffed Potato, Eggplant Parmesan and Italian Stir Fry With Linguini are all Spa favorites.

It is hard to beat steaming as a way to cook fresh vegetables to a tender crisp state. We steam almost all vegetables in the microwave. Follow the instructions in your microwave book, varying the time to suit your taste. We find that most vegetables are done in 4 minutes. For 2 servings of most vegetables, wash them and with water still clinging, put them in a glass dish, cover with plastic and microwave (high) for 4 minutes.

The more vegetables are processed, the more nutrients are lost . . . so minimize the cooking time as your taste permits and eat lots of vegetables for fiber, vitamins and minerals.

There are wonderful side dishes in this chapter. We sometimes combine several of them for a Vegetarian Medley. Vegie Rice Stuffed Peppers with a Carrot Flan or Cheese Stuffed Zucchini with Pasta Pesto make wonderful combinations.

Do include lots of fresh vegetables in your ULTIMATE RECIPE FOR FITNESS.

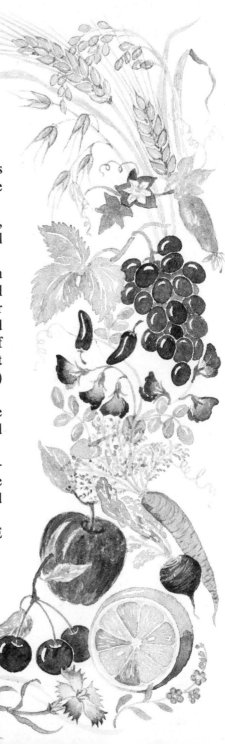

ARTICHOKE CHILI STUFFED POTATO

MAKES 6 SERVINGS   **180 CALORIES PER SERVING**

6   **POTATOES, BAKED**
         1. Split potatoes in half and remove most of the pulp. Leave just enough
         to help keep the skin intact.
         2. Set the potato pulp aside.

3 OZ.   **LIFETIME CHEDDAR CHEESE**
         3. Place in food processor and process to grate.
         4. Add the potato pulp and process to mix.

1/2 C. **GREEN CHILIES, CHOPPED**
1/2 C. **ARTICHOKE HEARTS, CHOPPED COARSELY**
         5. Fold into potato mixture and fill the potato skins with the finished product.

1/4 C. **LOWCAL SOUR CREAM**
1/4 C. **SALSA**
         6. Serve the potatoes topped with sour cream and salsa or let your guests help
         themselves to toppings.

NOTE: You might set up a bar with assorted toppings like guacamole, chopped olives, chopped scallions, grated cheese and chile beans. Everyone likes potatoes so let them star at your next party.

SHEILA'S FITNESS TIP: Hint for a healthy back — sit on the carpet or an exercise mat, keep your posture tall and straight, abdominals tucked in and wrap a towel around the sole of your foot. Hold the ends of the towel in your hands. Keep your left leg in a comfortable position. Now extend your right leg, keeping a slight flex to the knee and feel the stretch of your hamstring. Hold for a count of fifteen, release and switch legs. Repeat twice more on each leg.

CARB 30 GM (64%)   PROTEIN 9 GM (19%)   FAT 4 GM (18%)   SODIUM 58 MG

ASPARAGUS QUICHE

MAKES 8 SERVINGS   **120 CALORIES PER SERVING**

1 1/2 LB.   FRESH ASPARAGUS
1. Wash, remove and discard tough ends of asparagus.
2. Remove and save the tender tips of the asparagus for the top of the quiche.

2 1/2 C.   LOWFAT COTTAGE CHEESE (1%)
4 OZ.   LIFETIME MOZZARELLA CHEESE
1   SCALLION, CUT
1/2 C.   PARSLEY, FRESH
1   EGG
3   EGG WHITES
1 TSP.   HAIN NATURAL STONE GROUND MUSTARD
3. Combine in food processor and process to mix well.
4. Add tender asparagus stalks and process to chop, using an ON-OFF pulsing method.
5. Pour mixture into a nonstick sprayed quiche dish or pie pan, arranging the asparagus tips on top of the quiche. Asparagus must be covered with quiche mixture.

1 1/2 T.   GRATED PARMESAN CHEESE
6. Sprinkle over the top of the quiche and bake at 350 for 45 minutes until set and golden brown.

NOTE: This is excellent when baked and served in individual dishes and it freezes well. Enjoy this in the Spring when fresh asparagus is plentiful.

SHEILA'S FITNESS TIP: Set a realistic wellness goal. Instead of announcing to the world you are going on a diet, promise yourself that you will adopt a healthier eating pattern — less fat, sugar and salt and more high fiber foods.

CARB 5 GM (17%)   PROTEIN 17 GM (57%)   FAT 3 GM (25%)   SODIUM 374 MG

BRYANI (INDIAN RICE AND EGGPLANT)

1	TSP.	OLIVE OIL	1/8	TSP.	TUMERIC
1/2	TSP.	CUMIN	1/2	TSP.	CORIANDER
1/4	TSP.	CAYENNE	1/4	TSP.	CINNAMON

1. Heat spices in oil, stirring well.

3 C. EGGPLANT, PEELED AND DICED

2. Add Eggplant. Cook and stir until spices are absorbed.
3. Set aside.

1 C. BROWN RICE   2 C.   WATER
2 TSP. BERNARD JENSEN'S BROTH POWDER

4. Boil water, add rice and broth powder, cover and simmer for an hour until rice is tender.

2 C. GREEN BEANS, SLICED   1/4 C.   RAISINS
1/2 C. SCALLIONS, MINCED

5. Add to rice along with the cooked eggplant and bake at 325 for a half hour or to heat through.

1/4 C. ALMONDS, SLIVERED AND TOASTED

6. Serve Bryani topped with Almonds.

NOTE: This is a variation of a recipe taught by my favorite Vegetarian Cook, Dolores Ransome.

SHEILA'S FITNESS TIP: One out of every three exercise related injuries involves the largest joint in the body, the knee. To reduce the risk of knee injury, strengthen the muscles on the front of the thigh, the quadriceps. Sitting on a high stool, extend one leg slowly — hold for six seconds and lower the leg. Repeat ten times on each side.

CARB 18 GM (71%)   PROTEIN 3 GM (10%)   FAT 2 GM (19%)   SODIUM 3 MG

CANNELLONI

MAKES 6 TWO CREPE SERVINGS   **150 CALORIES PER SERVING**

12 CREPES (see BREADS AND MUFFINS)
1. Prepare and set aside

1	C.	**TOMATO PASTE**	2	TSP.	**GARLIC, MINCED**
1	C.	**WATER**	1/2	T.	**OREGANO**
2	T.	**OLIVES, CHOPPED**	1/2	T.	**BASIL**
1/4	C.	**HEARTY BURGUNDY**	1/2	TSP.	**THYME**
1/2	C.	**ONION, CHOPPED**	1/2	TSP.	**MARJORAM**
1/2	C.	**BELL PEPPER, CHOPPED**			

2. Combine in a sauce pan and simmer for an hour for sauce.

2 C. LOWFAT COTTAGE CHEESE (1%)   **2 T. GRATED PARMESAN CHEESE**
3 OZ. LIFETIME MOZZARELLA CHEESE
3. Combine in a food processor and process smooth.

2 T. SCALLIONS, MINCED   **1/4 C. FRESH PARSLEY, MINCED**
4. Add to food processor and process to mix for filling.
5. Place about 3 tablespoons of filling on each crepe and roll.
6. Put two crepes in each of 6 individual baking dishes, top with 1/4 cup of sauce and bake at 350 for about 20 minutes to heat through and melt cheese.

2 T. GRATED PARMESAN CHEESE   **2. T. PARSLEY, CHOPPED**
7. Serve with a sprinkle of parsley and cheese.

NOTE: This has been a guest favorite at The Oaks and The Palms for years. Your guests are sure to love it too! You will have some left over sauce which you can save to serve on pasta.

SHEILA'S FITNESS TIP: Moderate activity every day will do something positive for your heart.

CARB 12 GM (33%)   PROTEIN 17 GM (45%)   FAT 4 GM (21%)   SODIUM 382 MG

CARROT FLAN

MAKES 8 SERVINGS   **50 CALORIES PER SERVING**

1 LB. CARROTS, SCRUBBED AND SLICED
1/2 TSP. HONEY
1 TSP. BERNARD JENSEN'S BROTH POWDER
        WATER, TO COVER

> 1.Combine in sauce pan and cook until carrots are tender and water evaporates.
> TO MICROWAVE: Rinse, cut carrots and place in a covered glass bowl with the water clinging to the carrots. Microwave for 12 to 14 minutes until very tender.

2 T. BUTTER BUDS
1/2 C. EVAPORATED SKIM MILK
2 EGGS

> 2. Combine in blender with cooked carrots and puree.
> 3. Place in custard cups or individual ring molds.
> 4. Set containers in a pan of hot water and bake at 350 for 20 minutes or until custard sets.
> 5. Serve hot as a vegetable side dish in custard cup or unmold ring and fill with baby peas.

NOTE: This has been a favorite with our Oaks guests. They consider it worthy of a very special dinner party. Michael of Michael's Waterside Inn shared the original recipe with me and I left out the butter, the cream and the salt. Try that with some of your favorite high fat recipes. You might be surprised at how good you can make them taste.

SHEILA'S FITNESS TIP: Running or walking backwards helps strengthen the lower back, abdominals, hamstrings and quadriceps ... but don't do it alone. Get a partner and switch off. One of you moves backward, holding hands, when the other is moving forward. Switch off every five minutes.

CARB 6 GM (47%)   PROTEIN 3 GM (25%)   FAT 1 GM (28%)   SODIUM 45 MG

CAULIFLOWER PUREE

MAKES 6 SERVINGS   **50 CALORIES PER SERVING**

5 C. CAULIFLOWER, CHOPPED
   1. Steam 10 minutes or until tender. TO MICROWAVE: Microwave
   in a covered glass dish for 4 minutes or until tender.

1/2 C. LOWFAT COTTAGE CHEESE (1%)
1 T. NONFAT YOGURT
2 T. PARMESAN CHEESE, GRATED
1 TSP. BERNARD JENSEN'S BROTH POWDER
1/8 TSP. DILL WEED, DRIED
   2. Combine in food processor and process smooth.
   3. Add warm cauliflower and process to puree.

1/8 TSP. PAPRIKA
6 SPGS. PARSLEY OR FRESH DILL
   4. Serve on a warmed plate topped with paprika and parsley or dill.

NOTE: This is an interesting way to serve cauliflower and even confirmed cauliflower haters like the flavor. (They might not even know what it is unless you tell them.) This looks very nice served on a dark green or purple cabbage leaf.

SHEILA'S FITNESS TIP: Why is jogging hard on your body? Because each time your foot touches the ground your body experiences an impact of up to three times your body weight. To reduce the chance of injury, run on a flat surface and take a walking break for five minutes every mile.

CARB 9 GM (44%)   PROTEIN 5 GM (41%)   FAT 1 GM (15%)   SODIUM 126 MG

CHEESE BLINTZES

MAKES 8 TWO CREPE SERVINGS   **115 CALORIES PER SERVING**

16   CREPES (see BREADS AND MUFFINS)
             1. Prepare crepes and set aside.

1 QT.   LOWFAT COTTAGE CHEESE (1%)
1 T.   BROWN RICE FLOUR
             2. Combine in a mixing bowl and mix lightly with a fork.
             3. Place 1/4 C. of mixture on each crepe and roll.
             4. Place filled crepes on a nonstick cookie sheet and bake at 350 to heat through . . .
             about 15 minutes, depending on how cold they are when you put them in the oven.

1 C.   SLICED OR MASHED FRESH FRUIT (BERRIES, PEACHES,
             MANGO, PEARS, ETC.)
1 TSP.   ARROWROOT
1/4 C.   APPLE JUICE CONCENTRATE
             5. Whisk arrowroot into juice and thicken by cooking and stirring in a sauce pan.
             TO MICROWAVE: Whisk into glass measuring cup and microwave one minute to
             thicken. If a thicker sauce is desired, do another minute
             in the microwave.
             6. Add fruit to sauce and top blintzes with the resulting jam . . . or top blintzes with
             SOUR CREAM and then with the fruit.

NOTE: This is a revised version of one of our early recipes with the calories and fat reduced. I think it tastes a great deal better and it is certainly better for you. Try these for Easter Brunch, a festive luncheon or even a light supper.

SHEILA'S FITNESS TIP: Dining out is a sensual experience. A fast food lunch won't satisfy your senses so here's a great idea: Prepare extra portions of this recipe and package it for lunch, get out of the office and find a quiet spot to eat in peace.

CARB 9 GM (33%)   PROTEIN 15 GM (56%)   FAT 1 GM (11%)   SODIUM 474 MG

CHEESE STUFFED ZUCCHINI

MAKES 6 ZUCCHINI HALVES   **35 CALORIES PER SERVING**

3   **ZUCCHINI (about 6" each)**
1. Steam for 2 minutes and cool.
2. Cut in half lengthwise and scoop out seeds. TO MICROWAVE: Place zucchini in a plastic bag and microwave for 2 minutes.

1/2   C.   **LOWFAT COTTAGE CHEESE (1%)**
1 1/2   T.   **PARMESAN CHEESE, GRATED**
1   T.   **SCALLIONS, CHOPPED**
1   T.   **PARSLEY, MINCED**
3. Combine, mix well and spoon into zucchini shells.

1   T.   **PARMESAN CHEESE, GRATED**
4. Sprinkle cheese over each serving.
5. Bake at 350 to heat through, melt cheese and brown.

NOTE: This works equally well as a side dish or as part of a medley of stuffed vegies. We sometimes serve this at the Spas along with a stuffed potato and a stuffed pepper or artichoke.

SHEILA'S FITNESS TIP: Using a computer to input data burns 1.8 calories per minute for an individual who weighs 150 pounds. If your 'data base' (i.e., your bottom) is broader that you'd like it to be, it's time for an aerobic exercise program. You need 40 minute sessions 4 days a week. Walking, swimming, biking, jogging or rowing are all excellent choices.

CARB 3 GM (35%)   **PROTEIN 4 GM (44%)**   **FAT 1 GM (21%)**   **SODIUM 116 MG**

EGGPLANT PARMESAN

MAKES 6 TWO SLICE SERVINGS   **155 CALORIES PER SERVING**

ITALIAN SAUCE:

1	C.	ONION, CHOPPED	1/2	TSP.	BASIL
1	C.	BELL PEPPER, CHOPPED	1/4	TSP.	MARJORAM
1	TSP.	GARLIC, MINCED	1	TSP.	OLIVE OIL
1/2	TSP.	OREGANO			

1. Spray a skillet with nonstick spray, add olive oil and cook herbs and vegetables until onion is tender.

1	C.	TOMATO PASTE	1/2	C.	HEARTY BURGUNDY
1	C.	WATER	1	T.	OLIVES, MINCED
1	C.	MUSHROOMS, CHOP HALF AND SLICE HALF			

2. Reserving the sliced mushrooms, add to skillet and simmer for one hour.

1 LG. EGGPLANT, SLICED IN 1/2 INCH PIECES (12 SLICES)

3. Using high heat, broil quickly on both sides.
4. Place in individual shallow baking dishes or one large dish.

6 OZ. LIFETIME MOZZARELLA, SLICED

5. Top each slice of eggplant with a slice of cheese, cover with tomato sauce and top with sliced mushrooms.
6. Cover the cheese with the tomato sauce.
7. Top the tomato sauce with sliced mushrooms.

1/4	C.	BREAD CRUMBS	1/4	C.	PARSLEY, MINCED
1/4	C.	PARMESAN CHEESE, GRATED			

8. Combine and sprinkle over the mushrooms.
9. Bake at 350 for 20 to 30 minutes to heat thoroughly.

Note: Serve with a Mixed Green or Pasta Salad and some Parmesan Pita Crisps.

CARB 16 GM (40%)   PROTEIN 15 GM (36%)   FAT 4 GM (24%)   SODIUM 150 MG

FRESH MUSHROOM FILLETS

MAKES 6 SERVINGS   **110 CALORIES PER SERVING**

2 C.   FRESH MUSHROOMS, COARSELY CHOPPED
1   SCALLION, MINCED
1/2 C. BREAD CRUMBS AND WHEAT BRAN MIXED
1 T.   PARMESAN CHEESE, GRATED
1 TSP. DRIED DILL
        1. Combine in a large bowl and mix well.

1   EGG, BEATEN
        2. Add to Mushroom mixture and mix well.
        3. Form 6 patties and saute on nonstick sprayed grill to brown and cook through.

6 OZ.   LIFETIME CHEDDAR OR MOZZARELLA CHEESE, SLICED
        4. Top each Fillet with a slice of cheese and heat to melt the cheese.
        5. Serve with potatoes and vegetables or with a bun and lettuce and tomato to resemble a hamburger.

NOTE: This recipe came to me from Alan Hookers famous Ojai Ranch House Restaurant. I decalorized it with his blessing. It is wonderful when it is prepared immediately before cooking. If you must prepare ahead, saute the patties and reheat on the grill right before serving. Mushrooms lose their juice and flavor if chopped and left too long.

SHEILA'S FITNESS TIP: Wondering how to increase your energy? Exercise at lunch by joining a local health club. Preview a club before you join by asking for a free, one-time workout session. If the club is too crowded, noisy, or inconvenient, find another.

CARB 3 GM (10%)   PROTEIN 14 GM (50%)   FAT 5 GM (39%)   SODIUM 138 MG

ITALIAN STIR FRY WITH LINGUINI

MAKES 6 SERVINGS   **130 CALORIES PER SERVING**

1/2 LB.	LINGUINI	1 QT.	BOILING WATER
1 T.	BERNARD JENSEN'S BROTH POWDER		

1. Combine and boil pasta until tender but firm (12-15 Min.) Drain and set aside.

1 TSP.	OLIVE OIL	1 TSP.	BASIL
1/2 T.	GARLIC, FRESH PRESSED	1 TSP.	OREGANO

2. Combine in a large skillet and saute herbs to develop flavor.

1 C.	ONION, CUT IN 1/2 INCH CUBES
2 C.	BELL PEPPER, GREEN, RED, AND YELLOW, CUT IN 1 INCH CUBES
1 C.	ZUCCHINI, SLICED 1/4 INCH THICK

3. Add to herb mixture and stir fry over high heat until colors of vegetables turn bright (tender crisp).

1/4 C.	DRY VERMOUTH	1 TSP.	ARROWROOT, ROUNDED

4. Combine and then cook and stir into vegie mixture to glaze and sauce the vegetables.

5. Add pasta and toss to mix.

1 1/2 C.	CHERRY TOMATOES, HALVED	2 T.	PARMESAN CHEESE, GRATED
1 T.	FRESH PARSLEY, MINCED		

6. Serve the Italian Stir Fry topped with tomatoes, parsley and cheese.

NOTE: Notice that this dish is 14% protein which is the amount generally recommended. Don't fall into the trap of thinking that vegie meals that do not contain a piece of meat are low in protein.

SHEILA'S FITNESS TIP: Swimming is a wonderful sport for children. Call the 'Y' and sign up the kids for swim lessons. Don't know how to swim yourself? Adult classes start almost every month and swimming will tone your entire body.

CARB 23 GM (72%)   **PROTEIN 4 GM (14%)**   **FAT 2 GM (14%)**   **SODIUM 44 MG**

LENTIL DAL

MAKES 16 SERVINGS   105 CALORIES PER SERVING

4 C.   LENTILS (IF YOU CAN REMEMBER TO SPROUT THEM THEY WILL
        COOK FASTER AND HAVE MORE VITAMINS)
3 C.   YAMS, CUBED
1 T.   GARAM MASALA
1 T.   CORIANDER
1 TSP. CUMIN
4 C.   WATER
1 T.   BERNARD JENSEN'S BROTH POWDER
        1. Combine, bring to a boil, lower heat and cook for one hour until lentils are tender.
        TO MICROWAVE: Combine glass bowl and cook for 15 minutes; stir
        and cook for another 15 minutes.
        2. Mash or puree some of the mixture and serve with an Indian meal.

GARAM MASALA

MAKES 3 TABLESPOONS

1 T.   CARDAMON SEEDS   1 TSP. BLACK PEPPERCORNS
1 INCH   STICK CINNAMON   1   BAY LEAF
1 TSP.   CUMIN SEEDS   1 TSP. CORIANDER SEEDS
1 TSP.   CLOVES
          1. Combine in coffe grinder or blender and process to produce a powdery mixture.
          2. Store in a tightly covered container and keep with your spices.

NOTE: This can be purchased in the spice section of some markets.

CARB 39 GM (73%)   PROTEIN 13 GM (24%)   FAT TRACE (3%)   SODIUM 50 MG

MIDDLE EASTERN RICE PILAF

MAKES 8 SERVINGS   **75 CALORIES PER SERVING**

1/3 TSP. PEANUT OIL
  1 TSP. FRESH GINGER, MINCED
  1 TSP. FRESH GARLIC, MINCED

> 1. Heat oil and saute ginger and garlic in a sauce pan.

  3   CARDAMON SEEDS
  1 TSP. CORIANDER
  1 TSP. CURRY POWDER

> 2. Grind together in mortar and pestle and mix with garlic and ginger.

  2 T.   RICE VINEGAR
  2 T.   LOW SODIUM SOY SAUCE
  2 T.   DRY SHERRY
  1 C.   BROWN RICE
  2 T.   RAISINS

> 3. Add to pan, mix well and heat through.

1 2/3 C. BOILING WATER

> 4. Add to pan, cover tightly and simmer for 1 hour until rice is tender.

NOTE: This can be part of a vegetarian meal served with tofu and stir fried vegies or simply stand alone as a side dish. See the recipe for lower sodium Oriental Sauce under DRESSINGS, DIPS AND SPREADS.

SHEILA'S FITNESS TIP: Remember, you can even eat healthfully at fast food places by asking for less... or no mayonnaise, less calories by skipping the cheese on your burger, less fat and sugar by passing on the milk shakes and substituting lemonade or ice tea.

CARB 19 GM (84%)   PROTEIN 2 GM (8%)   FAT 1 GM (08%)   SODIUM 3 MG

PASTA PESTO

MAKES 6 SERVINGS   **170 CALORIES PER SERVING**

12 OZ. **SPINACH FETTUCINI OR SPAGHETTI**
1. Cook and set aside.

1/2 C. **FRESH SPINACH (PACK TO MEASURE)**
1/2 C. **FRESH BASIL LEAVES, CHOPPED**
1/2 T. **FRESH PRESSED GARLIC**
1 1/2 T. **WATER**
2. Place in blender and process to liquify.
3. Heat a large skillet, add spinach mixture, bring to a simmer
and cook for one minute.
4. Add pasta and toss to heat through.

3 T. **GRATED PARMESAN CHEESE**
5. Serve on heated plates and top each serving with a generous sprinkle
of cheese.

NOTE: Chef David Del Nagro brought the idea for this great Pesto from the famous Ojai Ranch House Restaurant. Our Spa guests love it and always request the recipe.

SHEILA'S FITNESS TIP: Baby fat, the kind that hangs on after baby is born, is easier to burn off if you're involved in a fitness program. Sign up for a mom and baby exercise class or get together with another parent and walk briskly every day for 30 minutes. Start slowly and get your doctor's O.K., of course.

CARB 32 GM (76%)   **PROTEIN 6 GM (15%)**   **FAT 2 GM (9%)**   **SODIUM 4 MG**

POTATO POTPOURRI

MAKES 6 SERVINGS   **200 CALORIES PER SERVING**

6   POTATOES
1. Scrub and bake until done.
2. Cool, slit and scoop out potato pulp, saving half for thickening soups or whatever.

1/2 C.   LOWFAT COTTAGE CHEESE, (1%)
2 OZ.   LIFETIME MOZZARELLA CHEESE
2 T.   BUTTERMILK
2. Combine in food processor with potato pulp and process smooth.

1/4 C.   PARSLEY, MINCED
1/4 C.   CHIVES, MINCED
1/2 TSP. DILL WEED, DRIED
3 C.   COARSELY CHOPPED VEGETABLES, LIGHTLY STEAMED
3. Combine herbs and vegies and fold into potato mixture.
4. Stuff potatoes and return to oven to heat through.

3 OZ.   FRENCH CREAM OR LOWCAL SOUR CREAM (see DRESSINGS, DIPS AND SPREADS)
5. Serve potatoes topped with a tablespoon of topping and some chopped chives or parsley.

NOTE: Be creative in your choice of vegies to use in this dish and then serve the potato surrounded with extra vegies... steamed to tender crisp perfection! It looks beautiful and tastes even better.

SHEILA'S FITNESS TIP: Tired eyes? Your computer could be to blame. But before you rub them one more time, start some eye exercises. Every fifteen minutes, look up from the screen to an object the farthest from your computer. Focus on the object for a count of five, then return to your work.

CARB 15 GM (25%)   PROTEIN 39 GM (67%)   FAT 2 GM (7%)   SODIUM 232 MG

QUESADILLA GREEN CHILI & TOMATO

MAKES 6 SERVINGS   **137 CALORIES PER SERVING**

6   **CORN TORTILLAS**
              1. Wrap in aluminum foil and heat through in a 350 oven. TO MICROWAVE: Place in a plastic bag and microwave one minute to soften.

6 OZ.   **LIFETIME MOZZARELLA CHEESE, SLICED**
1/2 C.   **GREEN CHILIES (A SMALL CAN)**
              2. Place cheese and green chili on half the tortilla, fold the tortilla over and grill until cheese begins to melt.
              3. Turn tortilla and grill and brown the other side.
1 C.   **LETTUCE, SHREDDED**
1/2 C.   **CHOPPED TOMATO OR FRESH TOMATO CHILI SALSA**
6 T.   **LOWCAL SOUR CREAM (see DRESSINGS, DIPS AND SPREADS)**
              4. Serve quesadilla topped with the above or on the side.

NOTE: This delicious and easy Mexican version of a grilled cheese sandwich makes a wonderful quick lunch. If you can afford more calories, some sliced avocado or guacamole adds a lot of flavor. Serve it to guests with a choice of many toppings. BE SURE to use CORN tortillas. Flour tortillas are made with lard and you don't need the saturated fat.

SHEILA'S FITNESS TIP: Read a menu with your heart in mind. Don't be timid when it comes to your health, request low fat, low cholesterol, high fiber menus and your favorite cafe will soon get the point. The healthy customer is always right.

CARB 18 GM (51%)   PROTEIN 12 GM (34%)   FAT 2 GM (15%)   SODIUM 56 MG

RACLETTE

3 OZ. LIFETIME SWISS CHEESE
1. Slice cheese very thin and line nonstick sprayed baking dish with cheese.

1 LB. RED POTATOES (WHITE ROSE WOULD BE 2ND CHOICE)
2. Steam potatoes until tender.
3. Slice potatoes 1/4 inch thick and layer over cheese.
4. Cover baking dish with aluminum foil and bake at 350 for about 10 minutes to just melt cheese and heat through. TO MICROWAVE: Cover dish with plastic wrap and cook on high for 2 minutes.

2 T. LOWCAL SOUR CREAM (see DRESSINGS, DIPS AND SPREADS)
1 TSP. DRIED DILL WEED OR THREE TIMES AS MUCH FRESH DILL WEED
5. Serve topped with sour cream and a sprinkle of dill.

NOTE: This can be made and served in individual baking dishes and makes a satisfying meal paired with lots of fresh steamed vegetables. Its name came from a dish served after skiing in The Swiss Alps. Raclette Cheese is kept hot and melting by the fire and the lucky guests dip pieces of potato in the cheese and eat it out of hand.

SHEILA'S FITNESS TIP: Feel bottled up inside? Get educated . . . enroll in a dance class, an exercise class or perhaps Tai Chi at the local community college. You'll have fellow students to talk with, increase your activity level and reduce stress.

CARB 14 GM (60%)   PROTEIN 6 GM (25%)   FAT 2 GM (15%)   SODIUM 22 MG

SESAME TOFU STIR FRY

MAKES 8 SERVINGS   **235 CALORIES PER SERVING**

2 LB. TOFU, DRAINED
1. Cut in 1 inch cubes and place on several layers of paper towels to drain; top with more paper towels and a small bowl as a weight.

1/4 C.	LOW SODIUM SOY SAUCE	1/2 T.	FRESH GINGER, MINCED
2 T.	DRY SHERRY	1/2 T.	FRESH GARLIC, MINCED

2. Combine for marinade and pour over Tofu, first removing the paper towels. Set aside.

1 TSP. PEANUT OIL   **1 T. FRESH GINGER, MINCED**
1 T. FRESH GARLIC, MINCED
5. Heat oil in wok or skillet and cook garlic and ginger over high heat.

4 C.	ONIONS, HALVED AND SLICED	3 C.	MUNG BEAN SPROUTS
3 C.	CELERY, SLICED THIN DIAGONALLY	3 C.	MUSHROOMS, SLICED
3 C.	BROCCOLI, SLICED THIN DIAGONALLY		

6. Add to wok and stir fry over high heat, adding a splash of sherry as needed to prevent sticking.

1/2 T. ARROWROOT
TOFU AND MARINADE
8. Combine marinade and arrowroot and mix with stir fry. Cook and stir over medium heat to thicken sauce.
9. Lower heat to a simmer, add tofu, cover and heat for two to three minutes.

2. C. COOKED BROWN RICE
2 T. SESAME SEEDS, TOASTED (OR CASHEWS, ALMONDS OR WALNUTS)
10. Serve on heated plates layering rice, stir fry mixture and a sprinkle of Toasted Sesame Seeds.

CARB 43 GM (66%)   **PROTEIN 13 GM (20%)**   **FAT 4 GM (14%)**   **SODIUM 164 MG**

SNOW PEA & MUSHROOM STIR FRY

MAKES 6 HALF CUP SERVINGS   **30 CALORIES PER SERVING**

2 C.   **SNOW PEAS OR EDIBLE PEA PODS**
4 C.   **FRESH MUSHROOMS, SLICED**
        1. Soak snow peas in cold water and pull off any tough strings.

1 T.   **CANOLA OIL**
        2. Place oil in wok or skillet and heat.
        3. Add snow peas and stir fry for 2 minutes.
        4. Add mushrooms and stir fry for a minute or two.

2 T.   **LOW SODIUM SOY SAUCE or LITE ORIENTAL SAUCE**
        (DRESSINGS, DIPS AND SPREADS)
        5. Add and toss with vegetables to season.
        6. Serve on a heated plate as an accompaniment to an Oriental meal.

NOTE: Be careful not to overcook this dish. It must be prepared right before serving to be at its freshest best.

SHEILA'S FITNESS TIP: They say when you're at the end of your rope, tie a knot. I say take a walk. Regardless of how awful you feel, walking around the block, vigorously, will release some of the tension, reduce the adrenaline that is produced in stressful situations and make you feel like you can cope.

CARB 6 GM (70%)   **PROTEIN 2 GM (25%)**   **FAT TRACE**   **(5%) SODIUM 2 MG**

SPANISH LENTIL RICE PILAF

MAKES 16 SERVINGS   **105 CALORIES PER SERVING**

3	C.	ONION, CHOPPED	3/4 C.	BROWN RICE
1	T.	PRESSED GARLIC	1/2 C.	LENTILS

1. Spray a kettle with nonstick spray and cook and stir until onion is tender.

1	C.	TOMATO PASTE	1 T.	CHILI POWDER
2	C.	WATER	1 T.	JENSEN'S BROTH POWDER

2. Add to kettle, bring to a simmer and cook for one hour or until lentils and rice are tender.

4	C.	MUSHROOMS, QUARTERED
6	C.	BELL PEPPERS, CUT IN 1/4 INCH PIECES (USE RED AND GREEN)
4	C.	CAULIFLOWER, COARSELY CHOPPED

3. Steam until just tender and stir into pilaf (about 3 minutes).

3	C.	CHERRY TOMATOES, QUARTERED

4. Toss with pilaf right before serving.

NOTE: This can be used as a side dish or as an entree. It can be combined with any of the Mexican dishes and is as delicious as it is nutritious.

SHEILA'S FITNESS TIP: What should be the most valuable item in your desk drawer at work? Your walking shoes! Wear them to and from work, even if you drive, and you'll feel more energetic and more apt to exercise. A lunch time walk can put energy into your afternoon and do great things for your bottom line.

CARB 21 GM (77%)   PROTEIN 4 GM (16%)   FAT 1 GM (7%)   SODIUM 19 MG

SPINACH QUICHE

MAKES 8 SERVINGS   **160 CALORIES PER SERVING**

2 PKG. SPINACH, FROZEN
1. Thaw and place in a quiche dish or pie pan.

1/2 C. ONION, MINCED
2. Mix with spinach.

2 1/2 C. LOWFAT COTTAGE CHEESE (1%)
2 EGGS
2 EGG WHITES
2/3 TSP. OREGANO
2/3 TSP. BASIL
2 TSP. BERNARD JENSEN'S BROTH POWDER
3. Combine in blender or food processor and process smooth.
4. Pour over spinach to cover.
5. Bake at 350 for 45 minutes to set.

4 OZ. LIFETIME LOWFAT SWISS CHEESE, GRATED
6. Sprinkle over hot quiche and return to oven just long enough to melt cheese.
7. Serve with sliced tomato.

NOTE: Enjoy this for Brunch, Lunch or Supper. It freezes well so why not make two and feed your freezer for a noncooking meal.

SHEILA'S FITNESS TIP: Does your company have a sports team? If not, start a rumor and you'll have a team. Soft ball, racquetball, walking, hiking are excellent choices for office groups anxious to shape up and slim down.

CARB 12 GM (28%)   **PROTEIN 20 GM (48%)**   **FAT 5 GM (24%)**   **SODIUM 415 MG**

SWEET AND SOUR PEPPERS

MAKES 8 SERVINGS   **30 CALORIES PER SERVING**

4 C.   **BELL PEPPERS (RED, YELLOW AND GREEN)**
1. Clean, seed and cut into 1 inch squares.

1/2 C.   **RED ONION**
2. Mince and toss with peppers.

1 TSP.   **BASIL, DRIED**
2/3 C.   **PINEAPPLE JUICE**
1/3 C.   **BALSAMIC VINEGAR**
1 T.   **ARROWROOT**
3. Whisk together in a small sauce, heat and stir over low heat to thicken for sauce. TO MICROWAVE: Combine in a glass measuring cup and microwave for 2 minutes to thicken. Whisk and set aside.
4. Steam peppers for 2 minutes, toss with sauce and serve. TO MICROWAVE: Place peppers in a plastic bag and microwave for 2 minutes. Toss with sauce and serve.

NOTE: This is very good cold and keeps for several weeks in the juice which actually seems to pickle the peppers. Be careful not to overcook or you will lose the beautiful color of the peppers.

SHEILA'S FITNESS TIP: Do you realize you can reduce the calories of a lavish restaurant dinner by 250 with just a squeeze? . . . That is, by squeezing on lemon for your salad dressing instead of the high fat, high sodium selections on the menu . . . or simply dilute the dressing with that same good squeeze.

CARB 7 GM (76%)   **PROTEIN 2 GM (17%)**   **FAT TRACE**   **(7%) SODIUM 13 MG**

TOMATO CORN SPOON BREAD PIE

MAKES 6 ONE CUP SERVINGS   **118 CALORIES PER SERVING**

1/4	C.	ONION, MINCED	1/4	TSP.	CUMIN
1		GARLIC CLOVE, MINCED	1	TSP.	CHILI POWDER (OR MORE)
1	TSP.	BASIL	3	OZ.	TOMATO PASTE
1	TSP.	OREGANO	3	OZ.	WATER
1	TSP.	BERNARD JENSEN'S BROTH POWDER			

1. Combine and simmer 1/2 hour for sauce. TO MICROWAVE: Place in a glass bowl or cup and microwave 10 minutes. Sauce should be the consistency of catsup.

2	C.	CORN, WHOLE KERNEL, (FRESH OR FROZEN)
3	C.	TOMATOES, PLUM OR OTHER FIRM TYPE, DICED 1/2 INCH
1	C.	GREEN CHILIES, DICED 1/4 INCH

2. Combine, mix well and place half cup portions in individual baking dishes or put the entire mixture in a quiche dish.
3. Spread 1 oz. of sauce over corn in each baking dish or over the quiche dish.

1   **RECIPE FOR SPOON BREAD TOPPING (see BREADS AND MUFFINS)**
4. Pour over corn tomato mixture and bake as directed.

NOTE: This recipe evolved from an attempt to make a TOMATO CORN POPOVER. The popover refused to pop, but the SPOON BREAD TOPPING saved the day. I hope that you enjoy this as much as our Oaks guests do.

SHEILA'S FITNESS TIP: This year, choose an activity vacation. Hiking in New Zealand, horseback riding in Colorado, a Florida tennis camp are a few of the dynamic ways to spend time together and help your children to learn the value of fitness.

CARB 28 GM (83%)   PROTEIN 5 GM (13%)   FAT 1 GM (4%)   SODIUM 17 MG

VEGIE FOO YUNG

MAKES 6 SERVINGS   **55 CALORIES PER SERVING**

2		EGGS
3		EGG WHITES
1/2	TSP.	GINGER, GRATED FRESH
1/2	TSP.	GARLIC POWDER

1. Combine and beat lightly in a bowl.

2		GREEN ONIONS
1/2	C.	BELL PEPPER
1/4	C.	CELERY
1/4	C.	MUSHROOMS
2	C.	MUNG BEAN SPROUTS

2. Chop coarsely and mix into egg mixture.
3. Heat a nonstick griddle and spray with nonstick spray.
4. Form pancakes of the desired size. Smaller cakes are easier to handle.
We generally make them about three inches in diameter.
5. Cook the pancakes until firm and then flip them over to brown on the other side.
6. The vegetables should remain crunchy.

NOTE: These are easy to make and very good. However they do not reheat well. It is best to prepare them right before serving. They combine well with other Oriental dishes or stand up well as an entree. By adding crab, shrimp or lobster, you can create a wonderful Seafood Foo Yung.

SHEILA'S FITNESS TIP: Meditation is a stress reducer used by many. Some fit folks meditate while they are walking. They call it 'moving meditation.'

CARB 4 GM (30%)   PROTEIN 5 GM (39%)   FAT 2 GM (32%)   SODIUM 56 MG

VEGIE RICE STUFFED PEPPERS

MAKES 6 SERVINGS   **210 CALORIES PER SERVING**

6 OZ.	TOMATO PASTE	1 CLOVE MINCED GARLIC
1 C.	WATER	1/2 TSP. OREGANO
6 OZ.	RED WINE	1/2 TSP. BASIL
1/2 C.	ONION, CHOPPED	

1. Combine and simmer for one hour for sauce.

3   BELL PEPPERS

2. Cut in half, clean out seed and membranes and place in baking dish.

2 C.	BROWN RICE, COOKED	1 C.	LOWFAT COTTAGE CHEESE (1%)
1 C.	MUSHROOMS, CHOPPED	2 C.	SPINACH, CHOPPED
1 C.	ONION, CHOPPED	1 C.	SUMMER SQUASH CHOPPED
1 1/2 C.	SAUCE (Reserve some sauce for topping)		

3. Combine, mix well and stuff peppers.
4. Cover baking dish and bake for one hour at 350.

2 T.   PARMESAN CHEESE, GRATED
THE RESERVED SAUCE

5. Serve the peppers on a heated plate, topped with a spoonful of sauce and a sprinkle of Parmesan cheese.

NOTE: These are wonderfully filling and satisfying on a cold night.

SHEILA'S FITNESS TIP: Time to learn a new family sport...weekend walk trips. Drive to a National Park, an open area, or the beach and spend family time talking, walking and hiking. Outfit the kids with a fanny-pack, some healthful snacks and pure water. You'll not only encourage health habits but you'll generate some great memories.

CARB 39 GM (71%)   **PROTEIN 11 GM (21%)**   **FAT 2 GM (9%)**   **SODIUM 232 MG**

SUMPTUOUS SEAFOOD AND PERFECT POULTRY

In Spa Cuisine we only use white meat of poultry and seafood so the recipes in this book all fall into those categories. Seafood is not only low in fat and calories, it in now believed that certain fish oils help to lower cholesterol. Most health professionals recommend 2-3 servings of fish per week for optimum health.

Buy the freshest fish possible and take care not to over-cook. Fish poached in the microwave in wine or fruit juice is moist, delicious and requires no fat in its preparation. You will find several recipes using this method of preparation in the chapter. Poached Salmon, Red Snapper Oriental and Baked Sea Bass are some of our favorites.

Chicken Breast appears to have no limit to the ways it can be cooked and served. You will find it in this chapter with recipes from The Orient, Italy and Mexico. The seasonings in those cuisines are so flavorful that it becomes easy to eliminate salt.

Ground Turkey has been a great boon to Spa Cuisine. I have yet to find a recipe calling for ground beef that suffered from substituting ground turkey. It is best to buy it fresh and to make sure the skin has not been ground in with the meat. The Tostada Bar, Tamale Pie and Ground Turkey Stroganoff are favorites.

Most health professionals recommend that you keep serving sizes of all meats and fish to about 4 ounces and add more vegetables and whole grains to your meals. If you are not already eating this way, try it as you work toward your ULTIMATE RECIPE FOR FITNESS.

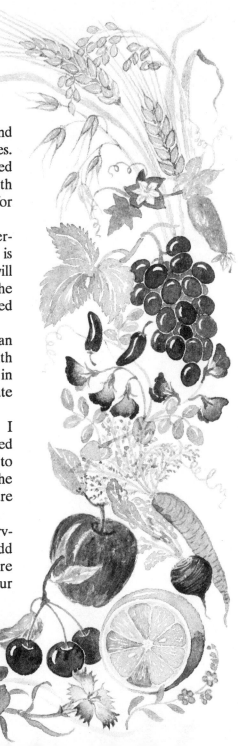

CANTONESE COCONUT CURRY CHICKEN

MAKES 8 SERVINGS   **190 CALORIES PER SERVING**

1 1/2 LB. CHICKEN TENDERS
　　　　　1. Cut into approximately one inch pieces and place in a bowl.

3 T. LOW SODIUM SOY SAUCE   **1/2 T. ARROWROOT**
3 T. DRY SHERRY
　　　　　2. Combine and pour over chicken to cover and marinate for 30 minutes.

1 TSP. PEANUT OIL
　　　　　3. Heat oil in wok or heavy skillet.
　　　　　4. Remove chicken from marinade, reserving marinade.
　　　　　5. Stir fry chicken until it is opaque, remove chicken and set aside.

2 TSP. FRESH GINGER, MINCED   **1 C. ONION, CHOPPED FINE**
1 T. GARLIC, MINCED   **DRY SHERRY**
　　　　　6. Stir fry ginger and garlic for about a minute, add onion and cook until translucent.

3 T. DRY SHERRY   **1 1/2 T. HONEY**
1 1/2 T. LOW SODIUM SOY SAUCE   **1 1/2 T. CURRY POWDER**
　　　　　7. Add to reserved marinade, stir into onion mixture and cook to thicken sauce.
　　　　　8. Return chicken to wok or pan to heat through.

2/3 C. NONFAT MILK   **2 TSP. ARROWROOT**
1 TSP. COCONUT EXTRACT
　　　　　9. Combine and stir slowly into sauce, cooking over low heat to thicken.
　　　　　10. Serve with brown rice and top with slivered almonds.

SHEILA'S FITNESS TIP: Want to avoid aches and pains? In a recent survey, it was proven that exercisers complain about them less — 55% versus 88% for non-exercisers.

CARB 20 GM (40%)   PROTEIN 18 GM (35%)   FAT 5 GM (24%)   SODIUM 88 MG

CHICKEN A L'ORANGE

MAKES 6 SERVINGS   **150 CALORIES PER SERVING**

1/4	TSP.	CARAWAY SEED, CRUSHED
1/4	TSP.	ROSEMARY
1	C.	ORANGE JUICE
1	TSP.	LOW SODIUM SOY SAUCE
1/2	C.	LEMON JUICE, FRESH
1	T.	ORANGE RIND, GRATED

1. Combine and place in baking dish for marinade.

6   CHICKEN BREAST HALVES, BONELESS AND SKINLESS (4 OZ.)

2. Place chicken in marinade, cover and refrigerate for 2 to 3 hours, turning from time to time.

3. Cover baking dish and bake at 350 for 45 minutes.

TO MICROWAVE: Microwave (high) for 10 to 15 minutes.

4. Drain off liquid into a sauce pan and keep chicken warm.

5. Boil liquid to reduce to one quarter volume for sauce.

6. Serve chicken with sauce spooned over to glaze.

NOTE: This looks lovely garnished with fresh Rosemary and Orange slices. If your sauce doesn't seem thick enough to cling to the chicken, thicken it with a little arrowroot. (1/2 T. to 1/2 C. sauce)

SHEILA'S FITNESS TIP: Condiments can fool you. Have margarine served on the side, dressing in a separate cup, tartar sauce in a little pot for dipping. You'll cut the calories and be able to taste the delicious, fresh foods you've chosen off the menu.

CARB 6 GM (17%)   **PROTEIN 23 GM (64%)**   **FAT 3 GM (20%)**   **SODIUM 50 MG**

CHICKEN CANNELLONI

8   **CREPES (see BREADS AND MUFFINS)**
1. Prepare and set aside.

1 LB. **CHICKEN BREAST, BONELESS AND SKINLESS**
2. Cut into 2 oz. portions and set aside.

1/3 C. **DRY VERMOUTH**   **1/2 TSP. BUTTER BUDS**
1 TSP. FRESH GARLIC, PRESSED
3. Place in a baking dish and heat to blend flavors.
4. Add chicken and turn to coat all sides with mixture.
5. Cover tightly and bake at 300 for half an hour to poach the chicken.

3/4 C. **LOWFAT COTTAGE CHEESE (1%)**   **2 T.   PAN JUICE FROM THE CHICKEN**
2 T.   **PARMESAN CHEESE, GRATED**
6. Combine in food processor and process to a sauce.

1 T.   **SCALLIONS, MINCED**   **1 T.   FRESH PARSLEY, MINCED**
7. Add to food processor and process to just mix.

1 C.   **ITALIAN SAUCE, (USE SAUCE ON PAGE 104 OR A SIMPLE SAUCE PAGE 133)**
2 T.   **PARMESAN CHEESE, GRATED**
8. Assemble the Chicken Cannelloni as follows. On one half of each crepe layer 1 oz. white sauce, 2 oz. of chicken and 1 oz. of Italian Sauce. Fold the crepe over and top with 1 oz. of Italian Sauce and a sprinkle of cheese.
9. Cover and bake at 300 for a half an hour to heat through.

NOTE: This is an easy dish to put together if you have crepes and Italian Sauce in your freezer.

CARB 5 GM (14%)   PROTEIN 22 GM (61%)   FAT 4 GM (25%)   SODIUM 231 MG

CHICKEN ENCHILADA

MAKES 12 SERVINGS   **180 CALORIES PER SERVING**

| 1 1/2 | LB. | CHICKEN BREAST TENDERS, | 1/2 | T. | GARLIC, MINCED |
| 2 | C. | ONION, CHOPPED | 1 | T. | SAFFLOWER OIL |

1. Saute together until onion is cooked.

| 1/2 | T. | CUMIN | 1/2 | T. | OREGANO |
| 1/2 | T. | BASIL | 1 | T. | CHILI POWDER |

2. Grind together in mortar and pestle and add to chicken.

| 2 | C. | TOMATO PASTE | 2 | C. | WATER |

3. Add to chicken, bring to a simmer and cook for an hour.

| 12 | | CORN TORTILLAS | 4 | OZ. | GREEN CHILIES, CANNED |

4. Soften tortillas by wrapping in aluminum foil and heating through in a 350 oven. (5-10 min.) Or heat in microwave in a plastic bag.
5. Fill each tortilla with 2 oz. (1/4 C.) of chicken and a strip of green chili, reserving sauce from chicken mixture.
6. Roll tortilla and place seam side down in a 9" x 12" baking dish or in individual baking dishes.

| 1 | PT. | BUTTERMILK |

7. Mix buttermilk with reserved sauce and pour over enchiladas to cover.

| 6 | OZ. | LIFETIME MOZZARELLA CHEESE CHEDDAR CHEESE, GRATED |

8. Top enchiladas with cheese, cover and bake at 350 for 30 minutes to heat through.

NOTE: These freeze beautifully, so make a lot and enjoy some noncooking nights.

SHEILA'S FITNESS TIP: Throw your scales away! It's measurements that count. Buy a pair of jeans in the size you look best in and never outgrow them.

CARB 22 GM (46%)   PROTEIN 14 GM (29%)   FAT 5 GM (25%)   SODIUM 396 MG

CHICKEN FAJITAS

MAKES 8 SERVINGS   **150 CALORIES PER SERVING**

1 LB.   CHICKEN BREAST (BONELESS AND SKINLESS)
1. Cut in strips and place in a shallow baking dish.

4 C.   RED AND GREEN BELL PEPPERS, SEEDED AND SLICED
2 C.   ONION, SLICED
2. Toss with chicken.

1/2 C.   TOMATO JUICE
1 TSP.   CHILI POWDER
1/2 TSP.   GARLIC POWDER
1 TSP.   ARROWROOT
1 TSP.   BERNARD JENSEN'S BROTH POWDER
3. Combine and toss with chicken mixture.
4. Place in a skillet, cover and simmer until chicken is cooked.
5. Remove cover and "stir fry" until sauce thickens and coats chicken and vegetables.

8   CORN TORTILLAS
6. Place in a plastic bag and microwave 2 minutes to soften the tortillas.

1/2 C.   LOWCAL SOUR CREAM (see DRESSINGS, DIPS AND SPREADS)
8. Serve the Fajitas in the tortillas with sour cream.

NOTE: Other condiments that go well with this meal are Salsa, Guacamole, Bean Dip and grated cheese. You will find recipes for the first three in the DRESSINGS, DIPS AND SPREADS chapter of this book. Put it all out and let your guests help themselves.

SHEILA'S FITNESS TIP: Write fitness into your date book. Make a date with yourself for that brisk walk at 8 A.M. When we commit ourselves to a project in writing, our chances of following through are considerably greater.

CARB 17 GM (45%)   PROTEIN 14 GM (35%)   FAT 3 GM (20%)   SODIUM 62 MG

CHICKEN WATER CHESTNUT MEATBALLS

MAKES 8 MEATBALLS   **25 CALORIES PER SERVING**

2	T.	SCALLIONS, CHOPPED
1/2	TSP.	FRESH GARLIC
2	T.	FRESH CUT GINGER

1. With food processor running, drop in all ingredients to mince.

3	OZ.	GROUND CHICKEN (OR TURKEY)
1/2	C.	FRESH MUSHROOMS
1	TSP.	LOW SODIUM SOY SAUCE

2. Add and process to just mix and chop mushrooms.

2/3	C.	WATER CHESTNUTS

3. Hand chop on cutting board to maintain texture and crunch.

4. Add food processor contents to cutting board and mix well, using your hands.

5. Form eight meatballs and place on nonstick sprayed cookie sheet.

6. Bake at 375 for 15 minutes to cook and brown.

7. Use in soup, stir fry or as an addition to any Oriental meal.

NOTE: These very light meatballs have a delightful crunch. Be sure to hand mix the water chestnuts to maintain texture and crunch.

SHEILA'S FITNESS TIP: Fit people feel less stress than those who lead a sedentary life. Why? Exercising brings a sense of control of body and surroundings. This continues into the work place and family situation. Start now with 'stress insurance' and exercise aerobically four times a week.

CARB 4 GM (54%)   PROTEIN 2 GM (28%)   FAT 1 GM (16%)   SODIUM 9 MG

COLD POACHED SALMON

MAKES 6 SERVINGS   **260 CALORIES PER SERVING**

6   **SALMON STEAKS (4 OZ.)**
6   **LEMON SLICES**
      1. Place salmon steaks in a glass baking dish and top each with a slice of lemon.

      WHITE WINE, TO COVER
      2. Pour the wine over the steaks and cover baking dish with aluminum foil.
      3. Bake 15 minutes at 350. The salmon should be opaque.
      TO MICROWAVE: Cover with plastic wrap and cook (high) 10-12 minutes.
      (Turn steaks after 5-6 minutes.)
      4. Cool in poaching liquid and serve on a chilled plate lined with lettuce
      leaves ... or serve it hot.

NOTE: At The Oaks we serve this with Tortilla Chips, PINEAPPLE SALSA (see DRESSINGS, DIPS AND SPREADS) and CUCUMBER CREME. To make the CUCUMBER CREME, combine the following in your blender and blend until smooth ... This is only 10 calories a tablespoon.

   1/4 C.   **CUCUMBER WITH PEELS AND SEEDS REMOVED**
     1 TSP.   **HAIN NATURAL STONE GROUND MUSTARD**
   1/3 C.   **LOWFAT COTTAGE CHEESE (1%)**
     1 T.   **LEMON JUICE**
     2 T.   **SCALLIONS**

SHEILA'S FITNESS TIP: Your teen may hate the thought of exercise, but don't discount the fact that surfing, skateboarding, biking and unorganized sports all contribute to strong adolescent bodies.

CARB 2 GM (6%)   **PROTEIN 27 GM (43%)**   **FAT 15 GM (54%)**   **SODIUM 108 MG**

CRAB CHABLIS

MAKES 8 SERVINGS   **134 CALORIES PER SERVING**

1 LB.   CRAB MEAT, CANNED, FRESH OR FROZEN
1. Rinse to remove salt and set aside.

4 C.   MUSHROOMS, SLICED   **1 T.   ARROWROOT**
2 C.   ONION, CHOPPED   **1 C.   CHABLIS**
2 TSP. HAIN STONE GROUND MUSTARD
1. Whisk wine, arrowroot and mustard together, pour in a skillet and heat to a simmer.
2. Add mushrooms and onion and stir over low heat to cook the vegetables and thicken the sauce.
3. Fold the crab into the mushroom mixture.
4. Place a generous half cup of The Crab Chablis in eight nonstick sprayed clam shells or ramekins.

1   C.   BREAD CRUMBS OR WHEAT GERM
2/3 C.   PARMESAN CHEESE, GRATED
5. Combine and sprinkle over crab to cover well.
6. Bake at 350 to heat through and brown topping.
7. Serve in the shells with artichokes, asparagus or a beautiful salad.

NOTE: This can be made ahead and reheated. It is definitely worthy of your favorite guests, but easy enough for family.

SHEILA'S FITNESS TIP: Did you know that housework, when performed in an active manner, burns 120 to 180 calories per hour, depending on your body weight and muscle to fat ratio. Remembering that could make cleaning house a lot more rewarding!

CARB 11 GM (34%)   PROTEIN 13 GM (31%)   fAT 4 GM (26%)   SODIUM 449 MG

FISH KABOB TERIYAKI

MAKES 6 SERVINGS   **105 CALORIES PER SERVING**

1/2	C.	LOW SODIUM SOY SAUCE	1/4	TSP.	FRESH GINGER, MINCED
1	TSP.	HONEY	1	T.	DRY SHERRY
1	TSP.	FRESH GARLIC, MINCED	1	T.	SCALLIONS, MINCED

1. Combine in a small sauce pan for TERIYAKI SAUCE.
2. Bring to a simmer, remove from heat and cool.

12		LARGE SHRIMP, PEELED AND RINSED
6	OZ.	HALIBUT, CUT IN SIX CHUNKS
6	OZ.	RED SNAPPER, CUT IN SIX CHUNKS

3. Place in a shallow dish and cover with TERIYAKI SAUCE to marinate for at least one hour.

12	PINEAPPLE CHUNKS, UNSWEETENED
6	RED PEPPER SQUARES (1 INCH)
6	GREEN PEPPER SQUARES (1 INCH)

4. Alternate on each of 6 skewers: 2 shrimp, 2 pineapple and one each of the peppers, halibut and snapper.
5. Broil for 5 minutes, baste with marinade, turn and broil to brown, basting as needed, about 5 more minutes.

NOTE: This is a delicious way to get one of the two or three servings of seafood that we need each week. For an easy, guest pleasing barbecue, put out an assortment of seafood in the marinade with cut up fruits and vegetables and let each guest assemble his own combination. The TERIYAKI SAUCE is also very good on chicken or lean beef.

SHEILA'S FITNESS TIP: Love beef? Order it occasionally in restaurants. Simply trim off all of the visible fat, avoid sauces and order it roasted or broiled.

CARB 5 GM (19%)   PROTEIN 17 GM (67%)   FAT 2 GM (14%)   SODIUM 75 MG

GROUND TURKEY STROGANOFF

MAKES 6 SERVINGS   **145 CALORIES PER SERVING**

1 1/4	LB.	GROUND TURKEY
1/2	C.	ONION, MINCED
1	C.	FRESH MUSHROOMS, CHOPPED
3/4	C.	BUTTERMILK

1. Combine, mix well and form into 6 patties.

2. Heat a nonstick skillet and grill until brown on both sides.

3. Remove and keep warm.

1 1/2	C.	MUSHROOMS, FRESH AND SLICED
1	T.	WHITE WINE

4. Add wine to skillet and heat.

5. Add mushrooms and cook until just done. Do not cook them until they shrink to half their size.

6. Top turkey patties with cooked mushrooms.

2	T.	SOUR CREAM, (see DRESSINGS, DIPS AND SPREADS)

7. Top each portion with a teaspoon of sour cream and serve on heated plates.

NOTE: If you don't have time to prepare the sour cream, use a purchased lowcal variety. Leftover patties are excellent when split and used on sandwiches or heated in sour cream and served over noodles.

SHEILA'S FITNESS TIP: Stress studies show that during exercise the brain releases a hormone called 'endorphine'. It makes you feel 'up'. Get high on this natural pep substance and — exercise away your problems.

CARB 4 GM (12%)   PROTEIN 25 GM (72%)   FAT 2 GM (16%)   SODIUM 133 MG

HOT SWISS TURKEY SALAD

MAKES 6 SERVINGS   **180 CALORIES PER SERVING**

2 1/2 C.   **TURKEY BREAST, COOKED**
1. Cut or tear into bite sized pieces and place in a bowl.

2 1/2 C.   **CELERY, SLICED**
1/2 C.   **ONION, MINCED**
2. Toss with turkey.

1/4 C.   **CREAMY MAYONNAISE (see DRESSINGS, DIPS AND SPREADS)**
1 TSP.   **LOW SODIUM SOY SAUCE**
3. Combine and toss with turkey mixture.
4. Place in a nonstick sprayed baking dish.

1/2 C.   **LIFETIME SWISS CHEESE, GRATED**
2 T.   **PARMESAN CHEESE, GRATED**
5. Top turkey mixture with cheeses and bake at 350 for 10 or 15 minutes to just heat through. Take care not to over cook. The celery should remain crisp.
6. Serve with steamed vegetables.

NOTE: You will never again wonder what to do with left over turkey. Everyone likes this and it couldn't be easier. If you don't have time to prepare the CREAMY MAYONNAISE, use commercial lowcal mayo and thin it down with buttermilk or lemon juice.

SHEILA'S FITNESS TIP: Set aside 15 minutes a day, just for you. This is your time to read, meditate, take a hot shower or stretch. This 15 minutes should be in addition to your regular exercise. It will be time well spent.

CARB 3 GM (7%)   PROTEIN 30 GM (70%)   FAT 4 GM (23%)   SODIUM 105 MG

ITALIAN TURKEY LOAVES

MAKES 6 SERVINGS   **100 CALORIES PER SERVING**

1 C.	ZUCCHINI	
3/4 C.	CARROTS	
1/2 C.	CELERY	

1/4 C.	ONION
1/2 T.	GARLIC

1. Wash and cut vegetables.
2. With food processor running, drop in the garlic to mince and then add the other vegetables to chop fine.

1 1/4 LB.	GROUND TURKEY
3/4 TSP.	MARJORAM
1 1/2 T.	BERNARD JENSEN'S BROTH POWDER

1/4 TSP.	THYME
3	EGG WHITES — 7

3. Add to mixture in food processor and process to mix.
4. Form 6 individual loaves on a cookie sheet.

ITALIAN SAUCE:

3/4 C.	TOMATO SAUCE
1/4 TSP.	OREGANO

1/4 TSP.	BASIL

5. Grind herbs in mortar and pestle and mix into tomato sauce.
6. Top loaves with sauce and bake at 375 for one hour.
7. Serve topped with fresh snipped parsley.

NOTE: These keep well, reheat well, taste good cold for lunch and just about everyone likes them. Even though they are half vegetable, they taste meaty.

SHEILA'S FITNESS TIP: Walking two miles a day, three days a week will add life to your years — not just years to your life.

CARB 56 GM (21%)   PROTEIN 11 GM (47%)   FAT 4 GM (32%)   SODIUM 60 MG

LEMON CHICKEN

160 CALORIES PER SERVING

1 LB. CHICKEN TENDERS

2 T. FRESH LEMON JUICE

1. Cut chicken in 1 inch pieces and squeeze lemon juice over them.
2. Cover and refrigerate for a half an hour.
3. Steam chicken for 10 minutes until tender and opaque.
4. Drain off juices from cooked chicken into a measuring cup. You should have 1/2 cup of juice. Add water if needed to make up the difference.

1 EGG

1 TSP. ARROWROOT

5. Combine with the half cup of juices in a sauce pan and stir over low heat to thicken the sauce.
6. Add the chicken to the sauce.

2 C. FRESH MUSHROOMS, CUT ABOUT THE SIZE OF THE CHICKEN PIECES

7. Add to chicken mixture and heat through. (Do this right before serving.)

2 C. COOKED BROWN RICE

8. Serve Lemon Chicken over brown rice on heated plates.

6 LEMON VERBENA LEAVES OR LEMON SLICES WITH PARSLEY SPRIGS

9. Use as a garnish.

NOTE: This dish has a lovely fresh lemon flavor.

SHEILA'S FITNESS TIP: Little ones love to stretch. After work, rent a yoga video and have fun and quality time. You'll relax and the little ones will thrive on the closeness ... with plenty of giggles thrown in for good measure.

CARB 17 GM (40%)   PROTEIN 16 GM (36%)   FAT 4 GM (24%)   SODIUM 77 MG

OVEN FRIED CHICKEN

MAKES 6 SERVINGS   **160 CALORIES PER SERVING**

3   SMALL CHICKEN BREASTS, HALVED AND SKINNED
1/2 C. ORANGE JUICE
1   T.   LOW SODIUM SOY SAUCE
         1. Place chicken bone side up and marinate for half an hour in a flat baking dish.

2   T.   PARMESAN CHEESE, GRATED
2 TSP. PAPRIKA
         2. Combine.
         3. Turn chicken breast side up and sprinkle with cheese mixture.
         4. Cover baking dish with aluminum foil and bake at 350 for 45 minutes.
         5. Uncover and bake for 10 to 15 minutes to crisp top.

NOTE: This is simple enough for your busiest days and tastes special enough to serve to company.

SHEILA'S FITNESS TIP: Before you consider medication to help with stress, take a vacation to a health resort. Sample all the programs, eat the low calorie food and pamper yourself. Make decisions about your job, lifestyle, and future when you're in a tranquil setting — not when you're sitting in 'gridlock' on Friday afternoon.

CARB 2 GM (6%)   PROTEIN 20 GM (50%)   FAT 7 GM (43%)   SODIUM 467 MG

PALMS CHICKEN SUPREME

MAKES 6 SERVINGS   **135 CALORIES PER SERVING**

3   **CHICKEN BREASTS (BONED, SKINNED AND HALVED)**
1. Slice each piece of chicken almost through and then open butterfly style.
2. Cover the open pieces of chicken with a piece of plastic wrap and pound lightly with a mallet until you have a flat, pliable piece of chicken. Keep covered and refrigerate.

1 T.   DRY VERMOUTH   **1/4 C.   ONION, CHOPPED FINE**
1 C.   SLICED MUSHROOMS
3. Saute mushrooms and onion in wine for 2 to 3 minutes.

1 T.   LEMON JUICE   **1 OZ.   LIFETIME MOZZARELLA**
1 OZ.   PARMESAN CHEESE, GRATED   **CHEESE, GRATED**
1 TSP. BERNARD JENSEN'S BROTH POWDER
4. Mix with mushrooms and onions for stuffing.
5. Place about 2 tablespoons of mixture on each piece of chicken and fold over.

1/4 C.   WHITE WINE
6. Pour the wine in a baking dish and set the stuffed chicken in the wine.
7. Cover tightly and bake at 350 for a half an hour.
8. Drain off pan juice and measure.

1/2 C.   PAN JUICE   **1 TSP. PAPRIKA**
1/2 T.   ARROWROOT
9. Combine in sauce pan and stir over low heat to thicken.
10. Serve chicken covered with a glaze of the sauce.

NOTE: This is very good served on a bed of brown rice.

CARB 2 GM (5%)   PROTEIN 23 GM (74%)   FAT 3 GM (21%)   SODIUM 134 MG

PARCHMENT BAKED SEA BASS

MAKES 6 SERVINGS   **200 CALORIES PER SERVING**

1/4	C.	MAYONNAISE (see DRESSINGS, DIPS AND SPREADS)
1	T.	LEMON JUICE, FRESH
1 1/2	TSP.	SCALLIONS, MINCED
1 1/2	TSP.	FRESH PARSLEY, MINCED
1/4	TSP.	DILL WEED, DRIED

1. Combine, whisk together and set aside.

1 1/2 LB.   SEA BASS, HALIBUT (OR WHATEVER YOU CAUGHT TODAY)

2. Cut fish in 4 ounce pieces and place each piece on a sheet of parchment paper.
3. Spoon a tablespoon of sauce over each piece of fish and wrap in parchment, crimping edges or double folding to seal tightly.
4. Place parchment wrapped fish in a baking dish and bake at 350 for a half an hour.

TO MICROWAVE: Microwave for 10 to 12 minutes, turning at half time.

NOTE: This is a favorite of our spa guests. We have had guests tell us that they had not found a better fish dish in the finest French Restaurants. And note how easy it is to prepare! The fish actually steams which requires no fat.

SHEILA'S FITNESS TIP: Fiber is the catch word of the 90s and broccoli is the magic high fiber vegie. Cup for cup it has more fiber than cabbage, string beans, spinach or cauliflower. There's evidence that fiber may be linked to the prevention of cancer in the digestive tract.

CARB TRACE (7%)   PROTEIN 29 GM (62%)   FAT 6 GM (31%)   SODIUM 292 MG

RED SNAPPER ORIENTAL

MAKES 6 SERVINGS   **100 CALORIES PER SERVING**

1 1/2 LB. RED SNAPPER FILETS
1. Cut into 4 Oz. serving pieces and place in a baking dish.

1   LEMON
2. Cut into thin slices and place a slice on each piece of fish.

1   BELL PEPPER, (RED OR YELLOW PREFERRED)
3. Wash, cut across, clean out seeds and membranes and place a cross slice of pepper on each filet.

1 1/2 T. SOY SAUCE, LOW SODIUM   **1 TSP. FRESH GINGER, MINCED**
1/4 C. DRY SHERRY   **3 T.   SCALLIONS, SLICED**
1   CLOVE OF GARLIC, MINCED
4. Combine, pour over Red Snapper filets and cover tightly with foil.
5. Bake in a 450 oven for 12 to 15 minutes.
TO MICROWAVE: Cover with plastic wrap and microwave for 6 to 8 minutes.
6. Serve on heated plates with an Oriental Stir Fry and some steamed brown rice.

NOTE: Even confirmed fish haters will like this and it just couldn't be easier. It can be put together early in the day and just popped in the oven before dinner. This is also very attractive done in parchment paper. Simply place each serving of marinated fish on a 12" x 12" piece of parchment paper. Fold and crimp edges to seal and proceed as above.

SHEILA'S FITNESS TIP: Don't reach for a cup of coffee or cola, instead do ten shoulder shrugs. Shrug your right shoulder to your ear and push it back down. Do five and repeat on the other side.

CARB 1 GM (6%)   PROTEIN 20 GM (85%)   FAT 1 GM (9%)   SODIUM 69 MG

RED SNAPPER VERA CRUZ

MAKES 6 SERVINGS

180 CALORIES PER SERVING

1 TSP.	GARLIC, PRESSED		1 C.	ONION, CHOPPED

1. Combine in a nonstick sprayed skillet and saute to wilt onion.

1 TSP.	BASIL		1 TSP.	CHILI POWDER
1 TSP.	OREGANO		1/2 TSP.	CUMIN
2 TSP.	BERNARD JENSEN'S BROTH POWDER			

2. Add to skillet and mix with garlic and onion.

1/2 C.	TOMATO PASTE		1 C.	WATER

3. Add to skillet, bring to a simmer and cook for 15 minutes.

1 1/2 LB.	RED SNAPPER, CUT INTO SIX PIECES

4. Place the snapper in a baking dish or 6 ramekins.

1 C.	CELERY, SLICED		1 C.	ZUCCHINI, SLICED
1 C.	WHOLE KERNEL CORN		1/2 C.	GREEN CHILIES
1 C.	RED AND GREEN PEPPERS, SLICED			

5. Toss together and place over and around the snapper.
6. Pour the sauce over all to cover and bake at 375 for 25 minutes.
7. Garnish with lemon and parsley.

NOTE: This is excellent with brown rice or the SPANISH LENTIL RICE PILAF (see VEGIES). This not only tastes good, it is a veritable feast of vitamins and minerals.

SHEILA'S FITNESS TIP: Do you know that roller skating burns about eleven calories per minute for the average size adult? It's excellent aerobic exercise, when done vigorously, and a splendid way to activate your kids.

CARB 20 GM (43%)   **PROTEIN 23 GM (50%)**   **FAT 1 GM (6%)**   **SODIUM 95 MG**

SALMON STEAKS IN COURT BOUILLON

MAKES 6 SERVINGS   **125 CALORIES PER SERVING**

1 1/2 LB. FRESH SALMON STEAKS   1 T.   PARSLEY, MINCED
    1 T.   LIME JUICE

    1. Place steaks in a skillet and sprinkle with lime juice and parsley.

1 1/2 C.   WATER   1   BAY LEAF
    2 T.   WHITE WINE   2   PEPPER CORNS
    2 T.   WHITE VINEGAR   1/2   CELERY STALK
    1   SPRIG PARSLEY
    1   CLOVE STUCK IN A SMALL ONION
  1/2 T.   BERNARD JENSEN'S BROTH POWDER
    1 TSP. HAIN NATURAL STONE GROUND MUSTARD

    2. Combine and simmer for 1/2 hour.
    3. Cover Salmon Steaks with hot liquid and simmer for 15 minutes or microwave.

    6   LEMON WEDGES
    6   PARSLEY SPRIGS

    4. Serve on hot plates garnished with lemon and parsley.

NOTE: The Court Bouillon or poaching liquid can be used for other firm fish. Since we are all trying to reduce our use of fat as much as possible, poaching has become a favorite way of cooking fish ... and your microwave oven can be your greatest time saver.

SHEILA'S FITNESS TIP: Don't be fooled by glamorous names. Ask your food server about ingredients and preparation. There is absolutely nothing wrong with turning down buttery sauces, creamy gravies and fatty batters. What do you get for being a health-conscious eater? About 300 fewer calories and absolutely great tasting food.

CARB 1 GM (3%)   **PROTEIN 17 GM (59%)**   **FAT 5 GM (39%)**   **SODIUM 328 MG**

SEAFOOD IN LEMON BUTTER SAUCE

MAKES 6 SERVINGS   **115 CALORIES PER SERVING**

6	OZ.	SHRIMP, PEELED AND RINSED
6	OZ.	SEA BASS, CUT IN SIX PIECES
6	OZ.	HALIBUT, CUT IN SIX PIECES

1. Place in a baking dish.

1/4	C.	BUTTERMILK
1	TSP.	BUTTER BUDS
1	T.	LEMON JUICE
1	TSP.	ARROWROOT

2. Combine and whisk until smooth.
3. Brush on seafood to coat.
4. Cover and bake 10 minutes at 350.
5. Uncover, brush with more sauce and bake 10 more minutes to brown.

NOTE: Before Butter Buds, we used to melt butter in buttermilk. This gives a butter flavor with a substantial saving in fat and calories. Easy and good!

SHEILA'S FITNESS TIP: Encourage your children to choose the fit life by your own example. If you sit and watch TV, if you drive rather than walk that half block or if you hire someone to rake those leaves, you're showing your kids that fitness isn't necessary. Change your values, if your health and that of your children is really important.

CARB 1 GM (3%)   PROTEIN 22 GM (80%)   FAT 2 GM (17%)   SODIUM 88 MG

SHRIMP ORIENTAL

2 C.	BOILING WATER	1 TSP. FRESH GINGER, MINCED
1 C.	BROWN RICE	2 TSP. FRESH GARLIC, MINCED
1 T.	LOW SODIUM SOY SAUCE	

1. Combine and cook over low heat until rice is tender.

1 10 OZ. CAN OF UNSWEETENED PINEAPPLE CHUNKS

2. Drain juice into a sauce pan, reserving chunks.

2 T.	WATER	3 T. APPLE CIDER VINEGAR
2 T.	HONEY	2 T. DRY SHERRY
3 T.	LOW SODIUM SOY SAUCE	1 T. ARROWROOT

3. Whisk the arrowroot into the sherry and combine all ingredients with pineapple juice in sauce pan; stir over low heat to thicken sauce.

1/2 C. BELL PEPPER, SLICED THIN   1/2 C.   ONION, SLICED THIN
1 C. TOMATO, SLICED THIN
THE RESERVED PINEAPPLE CHUNKS

4. Add to the sauce and keep warm.

1 TSP. PEANUT OIL
6 C. CHINESE VEGETABLES, CUT (BEAN SPROUTS, CELERY, ONION, CHINESE CABBAGE, SNOW PEAS, WATER CHESTNUTS, ETC.)

5. Heat oil and stir fry over high heat.

1 T. LOW SODIUM SOY SAUCE   1 LB.   LARGE SHRIMP, PEELED

6. Add to Chinese vegetables, cover pan and steam 2 to 3 minutes until vegies are tender crisp.

7. Serve rice, on heated plates, topped with vegies and shrimp with sauce spooned over all.

CARB 33 GM (51%)   PROTEIN 20 GM (39%)   FAT 33 GM (10%)   SODIUM 198 MG

SOLE WITH LOBSTER SAUCE

MAKES 6 SERVINGS   **115 CALORIES PER SERVING**

1 1/2 LB. **SOLE FILLETS (6 PORTIONS)** **2 T.** **WHITE WINE**
1. Place in a baking dish, cover and bake at 350 for 15 minutes. (Fish should flake easily.)
TO MICROWAVE: Cover baking dish with plastic wrap and microwave 8 to 10 minutes; rotate dish at half time.
2. While fish cooks, prepare the Lobster Sauce.

1/4 C. **ONION, MINCED**   **1/4 TSP.** **DRIED DILL WEED**
2 C. **MUSHROOMS**
3. Heat in a nonstick sprayed sauce pan.

1/4 C. **DRY VERMOUTH**   **1 TSP.** **ARROWROOT**
4. Combine, whisk smooth and stir into mushroom mixture.
5. Stir over low heat until mushrooms are cooked and sauce is thickened.

3 OZ. **LOBSTER, SHREDDED**   **1 TSP.** **FRESH LEMON JUICE**
6. Add to sauce, mix well and spoon over sole right before serving.

6 **PARSLEY SPRIGS**   **6** **LEMON WEDGES**
7. Garnish with beautiful sprigs of fresh parsley and the lemon wedges.

NOTE: Simple, delicious and wonderfully nutritious! What more could we ask. The fresher the sole, the better the results will be.

SHEILA'S FITNESS TIP: After enjoying the wonderful meals you have prepared from THE ULTIMATE RECIPE FOR FITNESS, you will probably find that your appetite has decreased. Why? One thing is that fat cells, as they shrink, send out chemical messages that trigger a decrease in appetite. No . . . your stomach does not shrink.

CARB 3 GM (7%)   **PROTEIN 24 GM (84%)**   **FAT 1 GM (7%)**   **SODIUM 22 MG**

TAMALE PIE

MAKES 8 SERVINGS   **180 CALORIES PER SERVING**

1	C.	ONION, CHOPPED	1/2	TSP.	DRIED OREGANO LEAVES
2		GARLIC CLOVES, MINCED	1/2	TSP.	CUMIN
1/2	C.	BELL PEPPER, CHOPPED	1	LB.	GROUND TURKEY OR CHICKEN

1. Combine in nonstick skillet and cook and stir until turkey browns.

1	C.	WHOLE KERNEL CORN
1/2	C.	OLIVES (SMALL, PITTED AND LOW SODIUM)
6	OZ.	CAN TOMATO PASTE
1	C.	WATER
1	T.	CHILI POWDER
2	T.	BERNARD JENSEN'S BROTH POWDER
1/4	C.	YELLOW CORN MEAL

2. Stir into meat mixture and mix well.

3. Pour into 1 Qt. casserole or quiche dish, cover and bake at 350 for 1/2 hour.

4	OZ.	LIFETIME CHEDDAR AND MOZZARELLA CHEESE, GRATED

4. Use to top Tamale Pie, cover and heat to melt cheese.

NOTE: This is really good and really easy. I sometimes do the whole operation in my Electric Skillet. If you have some extra time and can afford a few extra calories, try topping this with the SPOON BREAD TOPPING in BREADS AND MUFFINS. It looks and tastes spectacular!

SHEILA'S FITNESS TIP: If you haven't tried a new fitness activity in a year, you're over due. Rent a video about a different sport, see if you like the looks of it, then take lessons. Golf, basketball, karate, ballet... all are fun and you'll meet some great people who have chosen the fit lifestyle and a sane way to handle stress.

CARB 19 GM (33%)   PROTEIN 24 GM (33%)   FAT 6 GM (26%)   SODIUM 76 MG

TOSTADA BAR

MAKES 12 SERVINGS   **170 CALORIES PER SERVING**

12 **CORN TORTILLAS**
1. Crisp in a 350 oven for 10 to 15 minutes to brown.
2. Leave them in the oven to cool to produce a crisper tortilla.

1 1/2 LB. GROUND TURKEY
3. Crumble into a nonstick sprayed skillet and brown.

1/4 C. ONION, CHOPPED
4. Add to turkey in skillet and continue cooking.

1 T.	**CHILI POWDER**	**1 TSP.**	**GARLIC POWDER**
1 T.	**OREGANO**	**1 TSP.**	**CUMIN**

5. Grind together in a mortar and pestle and add to skillet as turkey and onion cook. Mix well.
TO MICROWAVE: Combine the preceding ingredients in a microwave safe casserole instead of a skillet. Cover and microwave for 5 minutes. Remove, stir and add the following 3 ingredients. Cover and microwave for 5 more minutes.

1 C.	**TOMATO PASTE**	**1 C.**	**WATER**
1 T.	**BERNARD JENSEN'S BROTH POWDER**		

6. Add to skillet and simmer 5 to 10 minutes.

4 C.	**LETTUCE, SHREDDED**	**1 C.**	**GUACAMOLE**
2 C.	**FRESH TOMATO, CHOPPED**	**1 C.**	**LOWCAL SOUR CREAM**
1 C.	**FRESH TOMATO CHILI SALSA**		**THE CRISPED TORTILLAS**
6 OZ.	**LIFETIME CHEDDAR CHEESE, GRATED**		**THE MEAT SAUCE**

7. Arrange in your most colorful pottery and let your guests create their own Tostada.

NOTE: This is the world's easiest way to entertain. Your guests feel that you have prepared a very special treat and you get to enjoy your own party.

CARB 7 GM (17%)   **PROTEIN 26 GM (60%)**   **FAT 4 GM (23%)**   **SODIUM 86 MG**

TURBAN OF HALIBUT

MAKES 6 SERVINGS

1 1/2 LB.   FRESH SPINACH, CLEANED AND CHOPPED WITH STEMS REMOVED
1/4 C.   ONION, MINCED
1/8 TSP.   DRIED DILL WEED
       1. Combine and steam or microwave 3-4 minutes to wilt the spinach.
       2. Set aside.

1 C.   LOWCAL MAYONNAISE
1 T.   FRESH LEMON JUICE
1 T.   CHIVES, MINCED
1 T.   PARSLEY, MINCED
1 TSP.   HAIN STONE GROUND MUSTARD
       3. Combine for sauce and mix half with spinach for filling.

1 1/2 LB.   HALIBUT FILLETS (OR SOLE AS THIN AS YOU CAN FIND)
       4. Spread 1/4 C. of spinach mixture on each fillet and roll securing with a tooth pick.
       5. Bake at 350 for 20 minutes.
       6. Serve turbans halved and set upright. The cut side will give you a firm base.
       7. Serve the extra sauce on the side.

NOTE: This looks absolutely elegant served on lightly steamed chard or kale leaves. Be careful not to overcook the spinach lest it lose its fresh green color.

SHEILA'S FITNESS TIP: When you order seafood in a restaurant, ask how it is to be prepared. Avoid those fried, broiled in butter and rich sauces. If you ask to have it broiled dry it will probably taste dry. Any chef can poach fish with no fat at all and it will be moist and delicious.

CARB 5 GM (12%)   PROTEIN 30 GM (69%)   FAT 4 GM (19%)   SODIUM 240 MG

TURKEY KABOB TERIYAKI

MAKES 6 SERVINGS   **175 CALORIES PER SERVING**

1	LB.	**BONELESS, SKINLESS TURKEY BREAST**

1. Cut into 1 inch cubes.

2	T.	**LOW SODIUM SOY SAUCE**
2	T.	**SHERRY**
1	TSP.	**MINCED GARLIC**
1	TSP.	**FRESH GINGER, GRATED**

2. Combine in a shallow dish and mix well.

3. Add turkey cubes, cover and refrigerate for one hour.

4. Turn turkey to marinate the other side and refrigerate for another hour.

1	C.	**PINEAPPLE CHUNKS, CUT IN ONE INCH SQUARES**
1/4	C.	**RED ONION, CUT IN ONE INCH SQUARES**
1/2	C.	**BELL PEPPER, (RED OR ORANGE) CUT IN ONE INCH SQUARES**

5. Blanch pepper & onion by placing in steamer for no more than 1/2 minute. Place immediately under cold running water to cool and stop cooking process.

6. Alternate 3 pieces of turkey with 2 pieces each of onion, pepper and pineapple on a skewer.

7. Broil or barbecue for about 5 minutes on each side, basting with the marinade.

NOTE: We sometimes place one inch chunks of potato on each end of the skewer. Use Red Potatoes with the skin on for some added color. For a fun barbecue party, set out the skewers with a variety of fruits, vegetables and turkey and let each guest choose their own combination.

SHEILA'S FITNESS TIP: Chinese food is ultra healthy, right? Unless you are careful, the answer is NO! Avoid fried shrimp, heavy sauces and fried rice and noodles. Enjoy the wonderful tender crisp chinese vegetables with steamed rice, chicken and seafood.

CARB 6 GM (14%)   PROTEIN 29 GM (67%)   FAT 4 GM (19%)   SODIUM 33 MG

TURKEY TOFU CHILI WITH BEANS

MAKES 12 SERVINGS   **215 CALORIES PER SERVING**

2 C. RED KIDNEY BEANS, DRIED
1. Soak overnight, drain and rinse.
2. Cover soaked beans with water, bring to a simmer and cook until tender. (2 to 3 hours)

1 LB. TOFU, FIRM
3. Freeze tofu and then thaw it, pressing out all of the excess water. Set aside.

1 LB. GROUND TURKEY   **1 T. PRESSED GARLIC**
2 C. ONION, CHOPPED   **1 T. CUMIN, GROUND**
1 TSP. OREGANO LEAVES, DRIED   **2 C. BELL PEPPER, SLICED 1/2 INCH**
4. Combine in a hot skillet and cook and stir to brown the ground turkey.
5. Add to cooked beans and continue to simmer.

1 C. TOMATO PASTE   **1/2 C. HEARTY BURGUNDY**
1 C. WATER   **3 T. CHILI POWDER**
1 T. BERNARD JENSEN'S BROTH   **1/2 C. GREEN CHILIES, CANNED**
POWDER
6. Add to beans with the tofu and simmer for a half an hour to blend flavors.

NOTE: Make a large pot of this and invite your friends or stock your freezer. We love a bowl of this topped with a bit of SOUR CREAM (see DRESSINGS, DIPS AND SPREADS) and Corn Tortillas, crisped in the oven. Add a green salad and dinner is served.

SHEILA'S FITNESS TIP: Eating in Mexican Restaurants can be a challenge! Choose soft corn tortillas with beans and/or Chicken Fajitas or a Tostada Salad. Watch those crisp Corn Tortillas; they get their crispness from being fried in fat.

CARB 32 GM (61%)   PROTEIN 9 GM (17%)   FAT 5 GM (22%)   SODIUM 19 MG

DYNAMITE DESSERTS

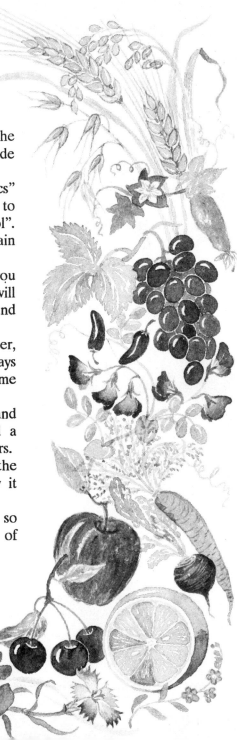

We are all born with a "sweet tooth" and it is often the lure of a serving of rich cheese cake or apple pie a la mode that prevents our achieving the slim figure we desire.

Many of our Spa Guests tell me that they are "chocoholics" or just can't resist cookies when they are hungry. The answer to that, of course, is to not let yourself ever get "out of control". If you are giving your body the food it needs, you will remain in control.

Make sure you get three servings a day of fruit and you may find that you are no longer a "chocoholic". The fruit will give you the sugar you crave. Follow Sheila's exercise tips and that too will help lessen food cravings.

Fruit not only gives us sugar; it also supplies us with fiber, vitamins and minerals. In this chapter, you will find many ways of serving fruit as a glamour dessert. You will also find some desserts combining fruit with yogurt.

For the days that you want something that seems rich and creamy, there are three Cheese Cake recipes, a Flan and a Trifle. When you long for pie, try the Fruit Tarts or Turnovers.

The Glazed Fruit is probably the most useful recipe in the chapter because it lifts plain fruits out of the ordinary. Try it once and it will become one of your favorites.

All of these desserts are low in fat, sugar and sodium so enjoy them as often as you like, perhaps incorporating some of them into your ULTIMATE RECIPE FOR FITNESS.

APPLE CUSTARD

MAKES 6 SERVINGS   **75 CALORIES PER SERVING**

3	C.	APPLESAUCE
1/2	T.	LEMON JUICE
1/2	T.	CINNAMON
1		EGG

1. Combine and mix well.

3		EGG WHITES

2. Whip until stiff.
3. Fold into apple mixture.
4. Divide mixture between 6 custard cups and bake at 350 to set custards.
5. Chill.

1/4	C.	NONFAT YOGURT
1	TSP.	APPLE JUICE CONCENTRATE

6. Combine, mix well and use as a topping for the custards.

NOTE: This simple, nutritious dessert is a great way to round out a fall dinner.

SHEILA'S FITNESS TIP: Vigorous exercise insures a vigorous sex life. In a survey of 160 swimmers, 40 to 80 years old, those most active in the pool were the most active in the bedroom, too.

CARB 14 GM (74%)   PROTEIN 3 GM (15%)   FAT 1 GM (12%)   SODIUM 39 MG

APPLE OAT CAKE WITH FRUIT CREAM

MAKES 24 SERVINGS   **70 CALORIES PER SERVING**

2 C. PIPPIN OR GRANNY SMITH APPLES
1. Core, quarter and steam for 10 minutes.
2. Place cooked apples and their juice in food processor and process to a sauce.

2 TSP. HONEY   **1 1/4 C. WHEAT BRAN, RAW**
1 T. LEMON JUICE   **1/2 C. NONFAT POWDERED MILK**
3. Add to applesauce and process to mix well.

1/2 C. OATMEAL
4. Add to apple mixture and process to just fold in, being careful not to over process and lose texture.

2 EGG WHITES
5. Whip until stiff, but not dry and fold apple mixture into whipped egg whites.
6. Spray a 9" x 13" baking pan with nonstick spray and pour batter into pan.
7. Bake at 350 for 30 to 40 minutes to brown.
8. Cool cake, cut into 24 pieces and top with ORANGE CREAM (this chapter).

NOTE: This is delicious 'as is' but if you can afford a few extra calories, toss in some chopped walnuts and dates or some raisins . . . SUPER GOOD!

SHEILA'S FITNESS TIP: Table tennis burns from 350 to 450 calories per hour—the same as brisk walking. Make it strenuous. Check your heart rate and have fun.

CARB 8 GM (57%)   **PROTEIN 5 GM (33%)**   **FAT 1 GM (10%)**   **SODIUM 82 MG**

APPLE TURNOVERS

MAKES 24 SERVINGS   **65 CALORIES PER SERVING**

8   FILLO DOUGH SHEETS
1. Follow the directions on the package. This means that you must plan ahead or forget this recipe as the thawing of the Fillo Dough cannot be hurried.

6 C.   APPLES, SLICED THIN (GRANNY SMITH OR PIPPIN)
2. Prepare and place in a mixing bowl.

2 T.   WHOLE WHEAT FLOUR
1/2 C.   APPLE JUICE CONCENTRATE
1 TSP.   CINNAMON
3. Combine and toss with apples to coat.
4. Working with two leaves of Fillo Dough at a time, cut in half, lengthwise.
5. Place a cup of the apple mixture across the end of each piece.
6. Roll like a jelly roll and place on a nonstick sprayed cookie sheet.
7. Continue until all Fillo Dough and apple mixture have been used.
8. Using a pastry brush, paint the top of each roll with the juice from the apple mixture, adding more apple juice concentrate if necessary. Sprinkle with cinnamon.
9. Bake at 375 for 12-15 minutes to brown.
10. COOL before cutting each roll in thirds.

NOTE: These freeze well so make a lot while you have some thawed Fillo Dough. You might also want to put some ONION SWISS TURNOVERS in your freezer for your next party. You'll find that recipe in the BREADS AND MUFFINS section.

SHEILA'S FITNESS TIP: Get the most from stair climbing and walk up that flight like Charlie Chaplin; knees flexed, pelvis tucked and WADDLE with a WIGGLE. Excellent for the inside of the thighs.

CARB 16 GM (89%)   **PROTEIN 2 GM (9%)**   **FAT TRACE (2%)**   **SODIUM 38 MG**

BAKED APPLE ALASKA

MAKES 6 SERVINGS   **55 CALORIES PER SERVING**

3		LARGE APPLES, HALVED AND CORED
3		DATES, PITTED AND HALVED
2	TSP.	APPLE JUICE CONCENTRATE
1/4	TSP.	CINNAMON

1. Place apples in a baking dish, brush with apple juice concentrate, sprinkle with cinnamon and place a half of date in the center of each apple.

2. Cover dish and bake at 350 for 45 minutes.

TO MICROWAVE: Use a glass baking dish, cover and cook for five minutes.

3. Uncover, set aside and cool.

2		LARGE EGG WHITES (ROOM TEMPERATURE)
1/8	TSP.	CREAM OF TARTAR
1	TSP.	HONEY

4. Beat egg whites to thicken and continue beating as cream of tartar and honey are added. Beat until egg whites hold stiff peaks.

5. Spoon pan juice over apples, top with meringue and bake at 450 for 5 minutes to brown the meringue.

6. Serve at room temperature within a half day.

NOTE: This will be easier to eat if you peel or score the apple, but you can eat the apple right out of the peel and then eat the peel which is very good. If you feel like spending a few more calories, you might add some raisins and/or walnuts to the date halves, but it is delicious as is.

SHEILA'S FITNESS TIP: 'Knock out' calves made easy. All you do is hold on to a counter and step up on a thick phone book with just the balls of your feet. Raise up, then release and lower heels toward the floor. Start with 10 and work up to 50 each day.

CARB 12 GM (85%)   **PROTEIN 2 GM (12%)**   **FAT TRACE (3%)**   **SODIUM 25 MG**

BANANA PINEAPPLE COCONUT RICE

MAKES 8 SERVINGS   **95 CALORIES PER SERVING**

1 C.   BROWN RICE, COOKED
1. Prepare the rice and cool.

1   BANANA
2 C.   PINEAPPLE
1/4 TSP. COCONUT EXTRACT
2. Combine in food processor and process smooth.
3. Mix with rice, place in sherbets or wine glasses and chill.

2 C.   MANGO, SLICED (OR PAPAYA OR PEACHES)
4. Arrange in a ring around the edge of each serving, leaving rice visible in the center.

1 T.   PALM SUGAR (AVAILABLE IN ASIAN MARKETS)
5. Top the rice with a light sprinkle of Palm Sugar.

NOTE: The idea for this nutritious dessert came from a recipe that was prepared in Don Skipworths Thai Class. His Sticky Rice Pudding with Mangoes was delicious but too high in fat and calories for Spa Cuisine. This is nutritious enough to eat for breakfast, (which I just did). The Palm Sugar has a very distinctive flavor so be sure to find it before making this dish.

SHEILA'S FITNESS TIP: Airline connection late? Use the time to de-stress and work out. Check your bag, slip into your walking shoes and briskly walk the entire airport until you feel slightly fatigued. Be sure to swing your arms and breath deeply and don't go near the escalator—only stairs are allowed on this program. The benefits? Normal travel inconvenience won't seem impossible and you'll feel great!

CARB 20 GM (89%)   PROTEIN 1 GM (6%)   FAT TRACE (5%)   SODIUM 3 MG

BANANA SPLIT

MAKES 4 SERVINGS   **65 CALORIES PER SERVING**

1   **LARGE BANANA**
               1. Cut in half and then in quarters lengthwise.
               2. Place two pieces of banana in each sherbet cup.

1/2 C.   **NONFAT YOGURT**
               3. Top each banana with 2 tablespoons of yogurt.

1/2 C.   **GLAZED FRUIT (RECIPE IN THIS SECTION)**
2 T.   **CAROB PEANUT BUTTER SAUCE (RECIPE IN THIS SECTION)**
2 T.   **ALMONDS, TOASTED AND SLIVERED**
               4. Top yogurt with 2 tablespoons of glazed fruit, a teaspoon of Carob Sauce and a teaspoon of almonds.

NOTE: This is nutritious enough to serve as the luncheon entree for a child's party. I sometimes mix the yogurt with some fruit sherbet which adds a few calories but is very good. The recipe as it is given here is the way we serve it at the Spas and I have never heard of anyone who did not enjoy it.

SHEILA'S FITNESS TIP: During exercise, allow your skin to breathe. If you must wear make-up, choose lipstick and mascara ONLY.

CARB 11 GM (63%)   PROTEIN 2 GM (14%)   FAT 2 GM (23%)   SODIUM 22 MG

BANANA WHIP

MAKES 3 SERVINGS   **25 CALORIES PER SERVING**

1   **MED. BANANA, CUT IN PIECES**
1. Place in a glass 4 cup measure and mash with an electric mixer.

1   **EGG WHITE, ROOM TEMPERATURE**
2. Add to banana and continue whipping until mixture is thick and holds soft peaks.

1 TSP.   **VANILLA**
3. Add and whip to mix well.
4. Spoon into dessert dishes and serve as a pudding or use as a topping as you would use whipped cream.

NOTE: Don't miss this recipe! It is so easy, so good and has so many uses that you'll be delighted. To make an absolutely delicious dessert for chocolate lovers, add a teaspoon of the CAROB PEANUT BUTTER SYRUP to each serving and give it a swirl...looks great and tastes even better.

SHEILA'S FITNESS TIP: After a workout, gently cleanse your body and facial skin, then apply a moisturizer. Allow it to be absorbed then blot off the extra. You may need a lighter moisturizer on your face and a richer one for dry skin areas like legs and arms.

CARB 5 GM (76%)   **PROTEIN 1 GM (21%)**   **FAT TRACE (3%)**   **SODIUM 17 MG**

BLUEBERRY MOUSSE

MAKES 6 SERVINGS   **50 CALORIES PER SERVING**

1 C.   BLUEBERRIES
1. Place in food processor and process to puree.

1/4 C.   APPLE JUICE
1 T.   GELATIN
2. Sprinkle gelatin over apple juice in a small sauce pan and let soften for 5 minutes.
3. Stir over low heat to dissolve gelatin and blend into blueberry puree with processor running.

2   LARGE EGG WHITES, ROOM TEMPERATURE
1/8 TSP. CREAM OF TARTAR
4. Combine and beat egg whites until soft peaks form.

1/4 C.   HONEY
5. Bring to a simmer, heat and stir for a minute.
6. Continue beating egg whites and slowly add honey.
7. Beat until egg whites hold stiff peaks and set aside.

1 C.   NONFAT YOGURT
8. Fold into fruit mixture and then into beaten egg whites.
9. Spoon into attractive glasses or sherbets and chill.

NOTE: This requires more steps than most of my recipes, but the results are truly spectacular. Other fruits, of course, may be substituted for the blueberries.

SHEILA'S FITNESS TIP: Warming up for exercise puts you in the right frame of mind and makes ligaments and tendons more pliable.

CARB 10 GM (76%)   PROTEIN 4 GM (23%)   FAT TRACE (1%)   SODIUM 18 MG

CAROB PEANUT BUTTER SYRUP

MAKES 16 SERVINGS   **15 CALORIES PER SERVING**

- **2 T.   HONEY**
- **2 T.   CAROB POWDER**
- **2 TSP. ARROWROOT**
  1. Combine in a small sauce pan and stir over low heat to blend.

- **3/4 C. HOT WATER**
  2. Add to carob mixture slowly and continue stirring until thickened.

- **1 T.   PEANUT BUTTER**
  3. Stir into syrup and remove from heat.

- **1 TSP. VANILLA**
  4. Stir into syrup and chill.
  TO MICROWAVE: Combine all of the above ingredients in a 4 cup glass measure or bowl, mix well and microwave for 2-3 minutes. Remove, whisk well and microwave for 1-2 minutes to thicken. Whisk again and chill.

NOTE: This is a marvelous mixture to keep in your refrigerator for chocoholics or anyone who likes the flavor of chocolate. We serve this as a dip for fresh strawberries and it is greatly enjoyed. This can also be used as a topping for ice cream, a dip for fresh fruit, or you can fold it into a whipped topping and serve as a mousse.

SHEILA'S FITNESS TIP: Fight a snack attack. Have a glass of water. It'll give you five minutes to decide if you truly need that treat.

CARB 3 GM (68%)   PROTEIN TRACE (7%)   FAT 1 GM (25%)   SODIUM TRACE

CARROT CAKE

MAKES 12 SERVINGS   **150 CALORIES PER SERVING**

2 C.   CARROTS
1. Place in food processor and process to chop fine.

2/3 C. WHOLE WHEAT PASTRY FLOUR	**1 TSP. VANILLA**	
1/3 C. BROWN RICE FLOUR	**1 TSP. CARDAMON, GROUND**	
2 T. HONEY	**1 T. ORANGE ZEST**	
1/2 C. APPLE JUICE CONCENTRATE	**4 EGG WHITES**	

2. Add to carrots and process to mix well.
3. Transfer mixture to a bowl.

1 C. DATES, CHOPPED	**1/2 C. WALNUTS, CHOPPED COARSLY**
2 C. ROLLED OATS	**1 TSP. BAKING SODA**

4. Fold into carrot mixture.
5. Pour into a 9" x 12" nonstick sprayed baking pan and bake at 350 for 40-45 minutes to brown.
6. Set aside to cool.
8. Serve cake topped with a tablespoon of the ORANGE CREAM (this chapter).

NOTE: At The Oaks/Palms we serve smaller portions of this and it is great success. Since it is a highly nutritious cake, treat your friends and children to a piece of this in the afternoon and watch that late afternoon slump disappear.

SHEILA'S FITNESS TIP: After you combine ingredients for this all-time favorite, add an energy booster. Step forward and clap hands above your head, step back and clap hands behind your back. Repeat 10 times then finish preparing this recipe.

CARB 18 GM (63%)   PROTEIN 4 GM (14%)   FAT 2 GM (23%)   SODIUM 10 MG

CRANBERRY APPLE CRISP

MAKES 14 SERVINGS   **70 CALORIES PER SERVING**

1/2	C.	APPLE JUICE CONCENTRATE
1/2	T.	ARROWROOT

1. Combine, whisk together, and stir over low heat to thicken. Mixture will be thick and clear.

TO MICROWAVE: Combine in a four cup glass measuring cup and microwave 2 minutes to thicken.

3	C.	FRESH CRANBERRIES, WASHED
3	C.	GRANNY SMITH OR PIPPIN APPLES, SLICED
1	T.	BROWN RICE FLOUR
1/2	TSP.	CINNAMON

2. Toss with apple syrup and place in a 9" x 12", nonstick sprayed, baking dish.

1/2	C.	ROLLED OATS
1/4	C.	GRAPE NUTS
2	T.	APPLE JUICE CONCENTRATE

3. Toss together to moisten cereal and sprinkle over Cranberry Apple mixture.
4. Bake at 350 for 40 minutes until hot and bubbly. Serve warm or chilled. FOR BLUEBERRY APPLE CRISP, substitute 3 cups of blueberries for the cranberries.

NOTE: This is a wonderful winter dessert. Top it with FRENCH CREAM, NONFAT YOGURT or LOWCAL SOUR CREAM. (DRESSINGS, DIPS AND SPREADS)

SHEILA'S FITNESS TIP: For fun and fitness, skip in place. Swing your arms, contract your tummy and breathe. Skip (or march if you prefer) to 100.

CARB 16 GM (89%)   PROTEIN 1 GM (6%)   FAT TRACE (5%)   SODIUM 15 MG

FITNESS FLAN

MAKES 6 SERVINGS   **110 CALORIES PER SERVING**

2		EGGS
2		EGG WHITES
2	C.	NONFAT MILK
3	T.	HONEY
1/2	TSP.	NUTMEG
2	TSP.	VANILLA

1. Combine in blender and process to mix well.

1 T. HONEY

2. Spray 6 individual custard cups with nonstick spray and put 1/2 Tsp. of honey in the bottom of each cup.
3. Place cups in 325 oven for 10 minutes to caramelize the honey.
4. Remove the custard cups from the oven and cool.
5. Put a half cup of custard mixture in each cup and then set the cups in a pan of water.
6. Bake for 45 minutes until firm and then remove and cool.
7. To serve, invert the Flan on a dessert plate.

NOTE: This is a revised version of an old favorite. The fat is reduced and the protein is increased by removing some of the egg yolks.

SHEILA'S FITNESS TIP: Exercise early in the morning. Regardless of how hectic or stressful your day becomes, you'll know that you've helped your body and mind cope better.

CARB 16 (57%)   PROTEIN 7 GM (26%)   FAT 2 GM (17%)   SODIUM 99 MG

FRESH APPLE JELL

MAKES 6 SERVINGS   **55 CALORIES PER SERVING**

1/4 C. **APPLE JUICE**
  1 T. **GELATIN**
       1. In a small pan, sprinkle gelatin over juice to soak.
       2. When all granules are translucent, stir over low heat to melt.
       TO MICROWAVE: Use a glass container and microwave for one minute.
       Stir until all granules are dissolved.

  2 C. **APPLE JUICE**
  1   **LARGE APPLE**
  1 TSP. **FRESH LEMON JUICE**
       3. Combine in blender and process to liquefy apple.
       4. Add gelatin mixture and blend well.
       5. Pour into 6 containers and chill to jell mixture.

NOTE: This has a lovely fresh apple taste and serves well as the conclusion to a heavy or spicy meal.

SHEILA'S FITNESS TIP: Prevent muscle soreness by increasing your workout (speed, weight or distance) by no more than 2 or 3 percent weekly.

CARB 14 GM (91%)   PROTEIN 1 GM (8%)   FAT TRACE (1%)   SODIUM 2 MG

FRESH FRUIT MIXTURES AS DESSERTS

MAKES 4 SERVINGS   **70 CALORIES PER SERVING**

TROPICAL FRUIT CUP

1/2	C.	FRESH PINEAPPLE, CUBED
1/2	C.	PAPAYA, CUBED
1	C.	BANANA, SLICED

1. Combine, toss together and serve one cup portions.

MINTED FRUIT CUP

4	C.	FRESH FRUIT, CUT INTO BITE SIZED PIECES
1	T.	FRESH MINT, MINCED
2	T.	LEMON JUICE
1	T.	APPLE JUICE CONCENTRATE

1. Toss together and serve one cup portions.

NOTE: Serve a fruit cup in a parfait or wine glass and it can be as glamorous as any dessert. Since few of us achieve the three servings of fruit a day that we should be eating, plan to use fresh fruit often in your meal plans. One last favorite of mine is a FRUIT KABOB. To prepare, simply cut wonderful fruit into bite sized pieces and thread on a skewer. How easy can it get!

SHEILA'S FITNESS TIP: A fresh fruit dessert has the plus of vitamins, minerals and fiber and is 300 calories less than a piece of fruit pie.

CARB 17 GM (90%)   PROTEIN 1 GM (5%)   FAT TRACE (5%)   SODIUM TRACE

FROSTED PEAR

3 MED. PEARS, FRESH AND RIPE
    1. Halve pears, remove seeds and place on a dessert plate, cut side up.

3/4 C. CREAMY CHEESE OR LOWFAT WHIPPED CREAM CHEESE.
1 T. SLIVERED ALMONDS, TOASTED
    2. Frost each pear half with CREAMY CHEESE (see DRESSINGS,
    DIPS & SPREADS) and garnish with a few slivered almonds.

NOTE: Doesn't it feel great to serve a dessert that looks attractive, tastes good and is also good for you?

SHEILA'S FITNESS TIP: Using an exercise video? Make sure you work at your own pace. Don't try to compete with the highly trained instructor or the models.

CARB 13 GM (81%) **PROTEIN 2 GM (11%)** **FAT TRACE (8%)** **SODIUM 44 MG**

FRUITED TOFU

1/4	LB.	TOFU, DRAINED
1		MED. BANANA
1/2	C.	PINEAPPLE, FRESH CUT

1. Combine in blender or food processor and process smooth for sauce.

1		MED. BANANA, SLICED
1	C.	PAPAYA, CUBED IN 1 INCH PIECES
1 1/2	C.	PINEAPPLE, CUBED IN 1 INCH PIECES

2. Place in a bowl and toss with tofu sauce.

3. Serve in sherbet or parfait cups garnished with a piece of the fruit and mint leaves.

NOTE: This extremely simple and highly nutritious dessert always rates raves and requests for the recipe. If higher water content fruits are used in place of the banana in the last three ingredients, the calories will be lower.

SHEILA'S FITNESS TIP: Side stitches occur often in those who are unfit. If you get one, inhale deeply, lean forward and press your fingertips into your side. Relax. Increase your program slowly because the adage of 'no pain, no gain' is a hoax.

CARB 18 GM (84%)   PROTEIN 2 GM (7%)   FAT 1 GM(9%)   SODIUM 2 MG

FRUITED YOGURT COMBINATIONS

MAKES 4 SERVINGS   65 CALORIES PER SERVING

2 C.   MIXED FRESH FRUIT (PINEAPPLE, PEACH, BANANA, BERRIES, ETC.)
1 C.   NONFAT YOGURT
1. Combine, mix well and taste; add a little honey or concentrated apple juice if needed.
2. Spoon into sherbets.

4   MINT OR LEMON VERBENA LEAVES
4   WHOLE BERRIES
2. Garnish with the above and serve.

YOGURT SUNDAE

Top plain non fat yogurt with fresh fruit.

NOTE: If you want to dress this up, use GLAZED FRUIT to top the yogurt and add a bit of CAROB PEANUT BUTTER SYRUP. Both recipes are in this chapter.

PEACH MELBA

Mix yogurt half and half with mashed banana and use to fill fresh peach or apricot halves . . . Top with a fresh raspberry.

FRESH FRUIT PARFAIT

Layer fresh fruit and yogurt in a parfait or wine glass. Glaze or sweeten the fruit as desired.

SHEILA'S FITNESS TIP: Did you know that jumping rope for 15 minutes burns about 125 calories for a 140 pound person? It's an excellent aerobic and fat reducing workout.

CARB 13 GM (74%)   PROTEIN 4 GM (4 GM)   FAT TRACE (4%)   SODIUM 44 MG

GLAZED FRUIT & VARIATIONS

MAKES 6 SERVINGS   **60 CALORIES PER SERVING**

1/2 C.   APPLE JUICE CONCENTRATE
2 TSP.   ARROWROOT
          1. Whisk together in a small sauce pan and cook and stir over low heat to thicken and clear.
          TO MICROWAVE: Whisk together in a 4 cup glass bowl or measuring cup and microwave to thicken (1 1/2 to 2 minutes).

4 C.   FRESH FRUIT (STRAWBERRY, PEACH, KIWI, MANGO, NECTARINE, BLUEBERRY, RASPBERRY AND PAPAYA ARE ALL GOOD CHOICES)
          2. Prepare fruit in bite sized pieces and toss with glaze right before serving.

CRANBERRY SAUCE OR GLAZE
2 C.   CRANBERRIES
          1. Add to the apple juice and arrowroot and cook until the cranberries pop.

JEWELED FRUIT SUPREME
          1. Spread the center of a pie plate with nonfat yogurt.
          2. Drop a teaspoonful of CAROB PEANUT BUTTER SYRUP in the middle of the yogurt and make a design drawing out from the CAROB SYRUP into the yogurt. (Use a toothpick for this)
          3. Arrange pieces of fruit over all and glaze. (CAROB PEANUT BUTTER SYRUP recipe is in this chapter.)

NOTE: If fruit is to be glazed as a topping, add the glaze after the fruit is placed.

SHEILA'S FITNESS TIP: Sledding, skating and cross country skiing are great winter sports and super calorie burners. A 150 pound adult can burn 500 to 700 calories each hour with these activities and when swimsuit season comes just watch out!

CARB 15 GM (94%)   PROTEIN 1 GM (4%)   FAT TRACE (2%)   SODIUM 1%

GLAZED FRUIT TARTS

MAKES 16 TARTS   **40 CALORIES PER SERVING**

16   GIOSO OR WON TON WRAPPERS
1. Place each wrapper between two small tart tins (1/4 cup) and press together firmly.
2. With a sharp knife, cut away excess dough.
3. Place on a cookie sheet and bake at 375 for 10 minutes. Remove the top tin and bake for 5 more minutes.
4. Remove and set aside to cool.

NOTE: Aluminum tart tins may be purchased in restaurant supply or gourmet cooking stores. This is such an easy way to make a great little tart shell with negligible calories (5 per shell), that it is worth while buying them.

4 C.   GLAZED FRUIT (RECIPE IN THIS SECTION)
1 C.   LOWCAL WHIPPED CREAM, BANANA WHIP OR NONFAT YOGURT
5. At serving time, fill each shell with GLAZED FRUIT and then add a tablespoon of the topping of your choice.

NOTE: For the calorie price of this recipe everyone can have 2 or 3 tarts. How about a Strawberry Tart, a Peach Tart and a Blueberry Tart. The cute little shells can also be used for puddings, whips or sorbets.

SHEILA'S FITNESS TIP: Exercise at a level that is right for you. Your fitness program should give you energy and not leave you exhausted.

CARB 9 GM (89%)   PROTEIN 1 GM (7%)   FAT TRACE (5%)   SODIUM 18 MG

INDIAN CHEESE CAKE

MAKES 12 SERVINGS   **100 CALORIES PER SERVING**

3   **GREEN CARDAMON PODS**
1. Remove seeds from pods and crush in mortar and pestle.
2. Place crushed seeds in a heavy pan over low heat.

2 C.   **LOWFAT RICOTTA CHEESE**
2 C.   **POWDERED MILK (NONFAT)**
3. Add Ricotta to pan and cook and stir, slowly adding powdered milk.
4. Continue to cook and stir to produce a smooth paste.

1 T.   **HONEY**
1 TSP. **VANILLA**
5. Add to milk mixture, heat and stir until it begins to dry.
6. Spread cheese cake on a parchment lined tray or dish and allow to dry for at least an hour.
7. Cut into 2 inch squares and serve garnished with tiny slivers of dried fruit.

NOTE: I decalorized this from an Indian recipe called BARFI. I had a feeling that the name might prejudice some so it became INDIAN CHEESE CAKE. The Cardamon gives this a unique and exotic flavor that most people find appealing.

SHEILA'S FITNESS TIP: People often consider martial arts as static routines, however, when performing martial arts, a 120 pound woman will burn about 650 calories per hour, while a 170 pound man will burn close to 800 calories per hour.

CARB 10 GM (37%)   **PROTEIN 9 GM (34%)**   **FAT 3 GM (29%)**   **SODIUM 57 MG**

LEMON PRUNES

1/2	LB.	PRUNES, DRIED
2		LEMON SLICES
		BOILING WATER TO COVER

1. Place prunes in a crock or bowl with lemon.
2. Pour water over the prunes, cover and refrigerate for at least four hours.
3. Serve as stewed prunes.

NOTE: This is one of our breakfast options at The Oaks and many guests have asked for the recipe. It couldn't be easier and the prunes swell up to twice their original size while the calories remain the same.

SHEILA'S FITNESS TIP: Ever wonder why ice hockey players are so trim? It's because the sport is a winner in terms of calories used. An hour of ice hockey for a 140 pound individual uses almost 875 calories. Combine that with a sensible, low fat diet and you know their SLIM secret.

CARB 25 GM (94%)   PROTEIN TRACE (4%)   FAT TRACE (2%)   SODIUM 1 MG

MANGO SORBET

MAKES 6 SERVINGS   **60 CALORIES PER SERVING**

2 C.   **FRESH MANGO MEAT AND/OR PULP**
1   **BANANA, PEELED AND CUT INTO CHUNKS**
1 C.   **PINEAPPLE PIECES**
         1. Freeze, place in food processor and process to a sherbet consistency.
         Reserve some fruit for a garnish.

1 T.   **LIME JUICE, FRESH**
         2. Add to sorbet and process to mix well.
         3. Serve in chilled sherbet cups and garnish with the reserved fresh fruit.

NOTE: This can easily be converted to a frozen yogurt by adding some nonfat yogurt to the mixture as it is processed. Make a wonderful PINA COLADA SORBET by leaving the mango out and adding a dash of Coconut Extract.

SHEILA'S FITNESS TIP: Six out of ten successful executives take time out during business hours to exercise or participate in sports.

CARB 15 GM (91%)   PROTEIN 1 GM (4%)   FAT TRACE (5%)   SODIUM 3 MG

MERINGUE SHELLS

MAKES 8 SERVINGS   *15 CALORIES PER SERVING*

4   EGG WHITES
1. Whip in a large bowl until foamy.

1/4 TSP. CREAM OF TARTAR
2. Sprinkle over foamy egg whites and continue whipping.

1   T.   HONEY
1   TSP.   VANILLA
3. Combine and add to egg whites very slowly as you continue whipping until the egg whites are stiff and form peaks.
4. Spray a baking sheet with nonstick spray and sprinkle lightly with rice flour.
5. Spoon 8 mounds of meringue onto baking sheet and form shells by making indentations with the back of a spoon OR if you have a cookie press with a meringue attachment, you can make very professional looking shells.
6. Bake at 250 for an hour or AS LONG AS IT TAKES for the shells to become crisp and crunchy. If they are soft, your recipe has not failed, you just have to leave them in the oven longer.
7. Turn the oven off and let the meringues cool in the oven.
8. Serve the meringues filled or topped with GLAZED FRUIT (RECIPE IN THIS SECTION), sorbet, or any of the other puddings or frozen desserts that you'll find in this chapter.

NOTE: These are easier than you might think and when you serve them to guests, they'll feel very special. If you have some left over and they turn soft overnight, you can crisp them in a 250 oven.

SHEILA'S FITNESS TIP: Regular exercise during a diet not only helps preserve muscle tissue that may be reduced by eating fewer calories but it allows the weight watcher to consume 25 percent more food than those on a diet-only plan (Peter D. Vash, M.D., U.C.L.A.).

CARB 2 GM (58%)   **PROTEIN 2 GM (52%)**   **FAT 0 GM (0%)**   **SODIUM 25 MG**

ORANGE CREAM AND CREAMY ORANGE PEANUT BUTTER

MAKES 8 SERVINGS   **15 CALORIES PER SERVING**

1/2 C.   **LOWFAT COTTAGE CHEESE (1%)**
1 T.   **ORANGE JUICE CONCENTRATE (OR APPLE OR PINEAPPLE)**
    1. Combine in food processor and process to blend well.
    2. Use as a frosting for cake or cookies or as dip for fruit.

CREAMY ORANGE PEANUT BUTTER   **(20 CALORIES PER SERVING)**

1/2 C.   **ORANGE CREAM**
1 T.   **PEANUT BUTTER (PLAIN GROUND PEANUTS, UNSALTED)**
    1. Combine in food processor and process to blend well.
    2. Use as a dip for apple slices, celery or carrots.

NOTE: When you buy peanut butter that has not been hydrogenated, you will often find oil floating on top when you open the jar. Pour the oil off and you will lower the calories and fat in the peanut butter. I sometimes turn the jar upside down on several layers of paper towels to drain off more fat. It leaves the peanut butter quite dry but that is ideal for the recipe given here. Peanut butter lovers who are afraid of the fat found in regular peanut butter love this recipe!

SHEILA'S FITNESS TIP: To reverse round shoulders which result from slumping over your desk or from bad posture habits: lace fingers overhead, bend elbows and gently push arms backward until mildly tight. Hold for a count of 30 and repeat 3 times.

CARB 1 GM (36%)   **PROTEIN 2 GM (54%)**   **FAT TRACE (10%)**   **SODIUM 57 MG**

ORIENTAL AMBROSIA

MAKES 8 CUP SERVINGS   **70 CALORIES PER SERVING**

2 C.   **PINEAPPLE, CUBED (FRESH IS BEST, UNSWEETENED CANNED O.K.)**
1 C.   **BANANA, SLICED**
1 C.   **PAPAYA, CUBED**
    1. Combine in a mixing bowl and chill.

2 TSP.   **COCONUT, SHREDDED AND TOASTED**
    2. Arrange fruit in attractive serving dishes and top with a pinch of toasted coconut.

NOTE: If you have some compatible fresh herbs such as mint or lemon verbena, they make a nice garnish for any fruit cup. Two dollars at a nursery and these plants, just stuck in a corner of your garden, will give you a constant supply. Any time you serve a fresh fruit dessert, you are giving your family and friends a nutritional plus.

SHEILA'S FITNESS TIP: A 154 pound person uses 5 to 10 calories a minute climbing stairs—heavier people use more calories, lighter people use fewer.

CARB 10 GM (89%)   **PROTEIN TRACE GM (4%)**   **FAT TRACE GM (8%)**   **SODIUM TRACE MG**

PASHKA (GREEK CHEESECAKE)

MAKES 24 SERVINGS   **60 CALORIES PER SERVING**

1	QT.	LOWFAT COTTAGE CHEESE (1%)	1/8	TSP.	ALMOND EXTRACT
1	C.	NONFAT YOGURT	1/2	TSP.	VANILLA
1/2	C.	POWDERED MILK (NONFAT)	1/4	C.	APPLE JUICE CONCENTRATE

1. Combine in food processor and process smooth.

1/2	C.	DATES, PITTED	1/4	C.	TOASTED ALMONDS

2. Add to food processor and process to JUST mix.
3. Line a new 8 inch flower pot with cheese cloth and pour in the cheese mixture.
4. Fold cheesecloth over the top and place a weight over that.
5. Place the filled, weighted flower pot on a plate and refrigerate for at least 24 hours to drain. (48 hours is better yet)
6. TO SERVE: Remove the Pashka from the flower pot, unfold the cheesecloth from the top and place upside down on a serving plate.

1/2 C.   FRESH STRAWBERRIES OR KIWI FRUIT

7. Garnish the Pashka with fruit and serve as part of a brunch buffet.

NOTE: This is a traditional Greek Easter dish. However, the original recipe used cream cheese, candied fruit and lots of nuts. We have been serving this as part of our Easter Brunch for quite a few years and always look forward to it as a special treat.

SHEILA'S FITNESS TIP: The longer the exercise session, even at lower aerobic intensity levels, the greater the metabolic-after-exercise effect. We sometimes call this the 'after glow' that continues to burn calories as you relax.

CARB 6 GM (39%)   PROTEIN 6 GM (43%)   FAT 2 GM (18%)   SODIUM 173 MG

PERSIMMON OAT COOKIES

MAKES 60 COOKIES   **40 CALORIES PER SERVING**

1	C.	PERSIMMON PULP
2		EGG WHITES
1/2	C.	APPLE JUICE CONCENTRATE
1	TSP.	VANILLA
3/4	C.	WHOLE WHEAT FLOUR
1/4	C.	BROWN RICE FLOUR

1. Combine in food processor and mix well.

1	C.	DATES, CHOPPED
1/2	C.	WALNUTS, CHOPPED
2	C.	ROLLED OATS
2	C.	CARROTS, GRATED

2. Combine in a mixing bowl.
3. Add persimmon mixture and mix well.
4. Drop by teaspoons on a nonstick sprayed cookie sheet.
5. Bake at 325 for 25 minutes.

NOTE: I like to bake these nutritious cookies in December when persimmons are plentiful in the Ojai Valley. If you don't have access to persimmons, substitute banana for a BANANA OAT COOKIE.

SHEILA'S FITNESS TIP: Muscle is more metabolically active than fat. The more muscles you have, the more calories your body burns when you're at rest.

CARB 6 GM (69%)   PROTEIN 1 GM (11%)   FAT 1 GM (20%)   SODIUM 2 MG

PUMPKIN CHEESE PIE

MAKES 6 SERVINGS   **75 CALORIES PER SERVING**

1 1/2	C.	PUMPKIN PUREE (OR WINTER SQUASH)
1 1/2	C.	LOWFAT COTTAGE CHEESE (1%)
1/4	C.	HONEY
1	T.	BLACK STRAP MOLASSES
1/2	T.	CINNAMON
1/4	TSP.	GINGER
1/8	TSP.	ALLSPICE
1/8	TSP.	NUTMEG
1		EGG YOLK

1. Combine in food processor and process to mix well.

3   EGG WHITES

2. Whip until stiff but not dry.
3. Fold pumpkin mixture into whipped egg whites and then into an 8 inch pie pan.
4. Bake at 325 for 45 minutes to an hour until firm.
5. Cool and refrigerate.

1/2   C.   SOUR CREAM or FRENCH CREAM (DRESSINGS, DIPS AND SPREADS)

6. Serve topped with one of the above from the recipes in this book.

NOTE: This can also be baked in individual custard cups. If you leave out the cottage cheese, you'll have CHIFFON PUMPKIN PIE which is also delicious. We sometimes serve it for Thanksgiving Dinner at The Oaks and our Thanksgiving Dinners are famous.

SHEILA'S FITNESS TIP: 300 overweight people who lost over 70 pounds and kept it off, have one thing in common...all increased their physical activity while reducing the amount of FAT that they were eating.

CARB 8 GM (40%)   PROTEIN 6 GM (33%)   FAT 2 GM (27%)   SODIUM 158 MG

RICE CAKES (FOR FRUIT SHORTCAKES)

50 CALORIES PER SERVING

1	C.	BROWN RICE FLOUR, SIFTED
1	C.	APPLE JUICE
1	TSP.	VANILLA
1/2	TSP.	ALMOND EXTRACT

1. Combine and mix well.

6		EGG WHITES
1/4	TSP.	CREAM OF TARTAR

2. Combine and whip to form soft peaks.

3. Fold rice flour mixture into whipped egg white.

4. Drop mixture into 12 nonstick sprayed muffin tins and bake at 350 for 30 minutes to brown slightly.

5. Turn out and cool.

6. Top the cakes with fruit or glazed fruit and whipped cream.

NOTE: Our Spa Guests are delighted when they find out that Spa Cuisine includes Strawberry Shortcake. However, the uses for these little cakes is limited only by your imagination.

SHEILA'S FITNESS TIP: A Stanford University study showed brisk walkers, runners and joggers, men and women ages 50 to 74, had stronger, healthier bones with 40 percent more calcium. Exercise is the right prescription for all who are concerned about osteoporosis.

CARB 10 GM (78%)   PROTEIN 1 GM (18%)   FAT TRACE (4%)   SODIUM 13 MG

ROCKY ROAD CANDY, SPA STYLE

MAKES 34 PIECES, (APPROX. 1 BY 1)   **12 CALORIES PER SERVING**

2	T.	HONEY	1 TSP.	VANILLA
1	T.	PEANUT BUTTER	2 T.	CAROB POWDER

1. Combine in a pan and cook and stir until melted.
TO MICROWAVE: Combine in a 4 cup glass measuring cup or bowl and microwave one minute. Stir until smooth. If mixture is too thick, add a few drops of water.

4   RICE CAKES, UNSALTED AND VERY CRISP

2. Break cakes into approximately one inch pieces in a non-stick large bowl.
3. Use a rubber spatula to scoop the Carob Syrup into the bowl and onto the broken rice cakes.
4. Use the same spatula with a fork to toss the mixture to partially coat the rice cakes.
5. Press the Rocky Road Candy into a nonstick sprayed eight inch pan or plate and cool.
6. Break or cut into one inch pieces and serve.

NOTE: Not too many people will stop at one of these if they have a chance to get more. However, you can eat four of them for under 50 calories. If these are left for a few hours or overnight, they will loose their crunch — to restore their crispness heat 1 minute in the microwave.

SHEILA'S FITNESS TIP: People over 55 who exercise regularly have better cognitive abilities than their less active counterparts (according to Drs. Louise Clarkston-Smith and Alan Hartley, researchers at Scripps College in Claremont, CA., and published in the Physician and Sportsmedicine).

CARB 2 GM (75%)   PROTEIN 8 GM (9%)   FAT TRACE (17%)   SODIUM TRACE

SHEILA'S CHEESECAKE DECALORIZED

MAKES 8 SERVINGS

80 CALORIES PER SERVING

3	C.	LOWFAT COTTAGE CHEESE (1%)
2		EGG WHITES
2	T.	HONEY
1	TSP.	VANILLA
1/2	TSP.	ALMOND EXTRACT
2	T.	LEMON JUICE

1. Combine in blender and process until creamy.
2. Place a pan of water in the bottom of a 350 oven.
3. Pour blender contents into a nonstick sprayed baking dish (9" x 12").
4. Bake at 350 for 45 minutes, reduce oven temperature to 300 and bake for 15 minutes longer.
5. Chill and serve alone or with glazed fruit.

NOTE: This has long been one of the favorite recipes at The Oaks and The Palms. However, something is missing in this newly revised version. It's the egg yolks. Leaving them out reduced the percentage of fat by over 20%. Reducing the calories, of course, allows us to have a larger piece. We often serve this with a glazed fruit topping. You'll find the recipe for the glazed fruit in this chapter.

SHEILA'S FITNESS TIP: Eating small meals during the day, instead of three big ones, may reduce your blood cholesterol level, reducing the risk of heart attack. A research group ate 17 snacks at hourly intervals for 2 weeks and lowered cholesterol levels 8.5% more than those eating the same amount and type of food in three normal meals. (Published in the *New England Journal of Medicine*).

CARB 7 GM (33%)   PROTEIN 11 GM (57%)   FAT 1 GM (10%)   SODIUM 357 MG

STRAWBERRY CHOCOLATE ECLAIR

MAKES 24 SERVINGS   **45 CALORIES PER SERVING**

24   POPOVERS (see BREADS AND MUFFINS)
          1. Prepare popovers and proceed as follows.

TO CREATE A STRAWBERRY CHOCOLATE ECLAIR:

1   POPOVER
1   LARGE STRAWBERRY
1 T.   BANANA WHIP, ORANGE CREAM OR FRENCH CREAM
1 TSP. CAROB PEANUT BUTTER SYRUP OR SYRUP FROM ROCKY ROAD CANDY
          1. Open Popover and fill with Whip or Cream of your choice.
          2. Add strawberry and top with Carob Syrup of your choice.

NOTE: Let your imagination be your guide in this. You might even put out Popovers with an assortment of fruit, whips, creams, and toppings and let people make their own.

SHEILA'S FITNESS TIP: Research proves people who view more than three hours of television per day are twice as likely to be obese as those who view less than one hour. (The Physician and Sportsmedicine)

CARB 5 GM (56%)   **PROTEIN 2 GM (23%)**   **FAT 1 GM (21%)**   **SODIUM 18 MG**

TRIFLE

MAKES 6 SERVINGS   **105 CALORIES PER SERVING**

1	T.	**GELATIN**
2	C.	**FRUIT JUICE (NOT FRESH PINEAPPLE)**

1. Soak gelatin in 1/4 cup of the juice and then heat and stir to dissolve.
2. When the gelatin mixture is absolutely clear, mix with the rest of the juice.
3. Pour into a glass bowl and refrigerate to set.

3		**RICE CAKES, MUFFINS, COOKIES OR CAKE (RECIPES IN THIS BOOK)**

4. Crumble and sprinkle over gelatin.

3/4	C.	**ORANGE CREAM (RECIPE IN THIS CHAPTER)**

5. Spread over crumbs.

1 1/2	C.	**GLAZED FRUIT (RECIPE IN THIS CHAPTER)**

6. Spread over ORANGE CREAM.

1/2	C.	**NONFAT YOGURT, FRENCH CREAM OR BANANA WHIP (THIS CHAPTER)**

7. Add dollops or lines of the above in any way you choose to form an attractive pattern.
8. Chill for several hours before serving.

NOTE: This SPA CUISINE version of an old English favorite has been an Oaks/Palms favorite for years. The original idea of the thrifty English was to create a sensational dessert out of leftovers. Vary the ingredients to suit your own leftovers and if you can afford a few more calories, sprinkle some toasted slivered almonds over the top just before serving. This can also be presented in individual sherbet or parfait cups.

SHEILA'S FITNESS TIP: A low fitness level is as important a risk factor for early death as smoking, high cholesterol, high blood pressure and family history of heart disease (*Journal of the American Medical Association*).

CARB 21 MG (79%)   **PROTEIN 5 GM (18%)**   **FAT TRACE (3%)**   **SODIUM 76 MG**

THE MENU FOR A TYPICAL DAY AT THE OAKS/PALMS

BREAKFAST: Our basic 200 calorie breakfast consists of a whole grain muffin, a high vitamin C fresh fruit and a vitamin and mineral pack. In addition, there are options, including oatmeal, shredded wheat and nonfat yogurt.

BROTH BREAK: POTASSIUM BROTH is served. (SENSATIONAL SOUPS)

LUNCH: Our 350 calorie lunch generally begins with soup, followed by an Entree Salad, Tostada, Crepes or Quiches with fresh fruit for dessert.

VEGIE BREAK: Assorted raw vegetables provide a refreshing pick up.

HAPPY HOUR JUICE: Fresh fruit blended into grapefruit juice is the beverage of choice.

DINNER: Our 350 calorie dinner begins with soup or salad, followed by a seafood, poultry or vegetarian entree and finishing with one of our more glamourous desserts.

EVENING SNACK: A cup of hot air popped popcorn or a cookie with herb tea ends the day. Notice that there are snacks throughout the day. It is so much easier to remain in control and enjoy food when we do not allow ourselves to get too hungry.

RECIPES FOR FITNESS FOR VERY BUSY PEOPLE has several chapters on getting organized to shop and cook for fitness. If you don't have it, there is an order blank in the back of this book.

See the following two pages for 4 weeks of dinner menus.

TWENTY-EIGHT DAY DINNER MENU

WEEK ONE

SUNDAY
Apple Cabbage Slaw
Chicken Enchilada
Sweet and Sour Peppers
Baked Apple Alaska

THURSDAY
Orange Zucchini Salad
Ground Turkey
  Stroganoff
Steamed Spinach
  with Onion
Glazed Fruit Supreme

MONDAY
Tomato, Basil
  Mozzarella Salad
Artichoke Chili
  Stuffed Potato
Mixed Steamed Vegies
Parfait

FRIDAY
Mixed Greens & Kiwi w/
  Raspberry Vinaigrette
Fish KaBob
Steamed Carrots
Apple Oat Cake

TUESDAY
Mixed Green Salad
Crab Chablis
Middle Eastern Rice
  Pilaf
Steamed Broccoli
Blueberry Mousse

SATURDAY
Sambals
Cantonese Coconut
  Curry Chicken
Middle Easter Rice
  Pilaf
Snow Peas/Mushroom
  Stir Fry
Indian Cheese Cake

WEDNESDAY
Antipasto Salad
Cannelloni
Parmesan Pita Crisp
Fitness Flan

WEEK TWO

SUNDAY
Spinach Salad
Chicken A L'Orange
Steamed Broccoli
Steamed Carrots
Apple Turnover

THURSDAY
Antipasto Salad
Chicken Cannelloni
Pasta Pesto
Fruited Yogurt

MONDAY
Mixed Green Salad w/
  Avocado Dressing
Eggplant Parmesan w/
  Garlic Toast
Strawberry Chocolate
  Eclair

FRIDAY
Oriental Cucumber
  Salad
Won Ton Crisps
Red Snapper Oriental
Mixed Pepper Stir Fry
Fruited Tofu

TUESDAY
Fresh Mushroom Salad
Parchment Baked
  Sea Bass
Carrot Flan
Baby Peas
Cranberry Apple Crisp

SATURDAY
Mixed Green Salad w/
  Italian Dressing
Italian Turkey Loaf
Spaghetti Squash
Green Beans
Trifle

WEDNESDAY
Carrot Date Salad
  w/ Walnuts
Fresh Mushroom Filets
Baked Potato
Sheila's Cheesecake w/ Glazed
  Kiwi

TWENTY-EIGHT DAY DINNER MENU

WEEK THREE

SUNDAY
Lettuce & Tomato
  Salad
Hot Swiss Turkey
  Salad
Popovers
Strawberry Shortcake

MONDAY
Costa Rican Tomato
  Soup
Chicken Fajita
Bean Dip
Lettuce & Tomato
Peach Melba

TUESDAY
Bibb Lettuce w/
  Raspberry Vinaigrette
Salmon Steaks in Court
  Bouillon
Cauliflower Puree
Steamed Spinach
Glazed Fruit Tarts

WEDNESDAY
Orange Zucchini Salad
Tamale Pie
Tortilla Chips
Pina Colada Sorbet

THURSDAY
Antipasto Salad
Italian Stir Fry with
  Linguini
Parmesan Pita Crisps
Banana Whip

FRIDAY
Mixed Greens with
  Avocado Dressing
Sole with Lobster Sauce
Raclette
Steamed Broccoli
Carrot Cake

SATURDAY
Oriental Cucumber Salad
Sesame Tofu Stir Fry
Brown Rice
Snow Peas
Oriental Ambrosia

WEEK FOUR

SUNDAY
Gazpacho
Tostada Bar
Mango Sorbet

MONDAY
Herbed Red Potato
  Salad
Asparagus Quiche
Lettuce with Sliced
  Tomato
Glazed Fruit Supreme

TUESDAY
Mexican Orange Onion
  Salad
Red Snapper Vera Cruz
Spanish Lentil Rice
  Pilaf
Banana Pineapple
  Coconut Rice

WEDNESDAY
Apple Cabbage Slaw Veronica
Lemon Chicken
Spinach Pasta
Mixed Steamed Vegies
Crepes w/ Glaze Fruit

THURSDAY
Mixed Greens with
  Italian Dressing
Vegie Rice Stuffed
  Peppers
Parmesan Pita Crisps
Pashka

FRIDAY
Marinated Beet and
  Onion Salad
Turban of Halibut
Baked Potato with
  Sour Cream
Green Beans
Banana Split

SATURDAY
Mixed Lettuce w/
  Buttermilk Dressing
Palms Chicken Supreme
Wild Rice Pilaf
Meringue Shells with
  Glazed Blueberries

INDEX

To order, check appropriate box (prices include tax and shipping):

...ks

New Favorite Recipes for Fitness"...........................$ 6.24
    By Eleanor Brown
Take 5"..$11.58
    By Sheila Cluff
The Ultimate Recipe for Fitness".............................$19.03
    By Sheila Cluff and Eleanor Brown
Recipes for Fitness for Very Busy People.................$10.23
    By Eleanor Brown

...ness Equipment

...ower Bands...$28.19
...ool Hand Paddles..$ 9.38
...ick Board for the Pool......................................$ 9.89
...ater Woggles..$ 8.59
...lex-A-Ball (Includes video and brochure)..............$35.12

...ks' and Palms' Custom Blends

..."Warming" Essential Massage Oil.........................$15.00
..."Tranquility" Essential Massage Oil......................$15.00
..."Restorative" Essential Massage Oil......................$15.00
..."Cleansing & Toning" Essential Massage Oil...........$15.00
...Aromatherapy Body Lotion.................................$16.00
...Lavender Hydrosol Mist.....................................$15.00
...Orange Hydrosol Mist.......................................$15.00
...Rose Hydrosol Mist..$15.00
...Mineral Salt for Salt Glo Treatment......................$15.00

...mpering Products

...Herbal Eye Pillow...$17.00
...Warming Booties and Mittens..............................$42.95
...White 3/4 length Cotton Waffle Bathrobes w/ Oaks or Palms
    logo..$47.00

Seasoning

__ Dr. Bernard Jensen's Broth/Seasoning Powder...............$11.50
__ Dad's Italian Seasoning......................................$ 8.95

Spa Workout Audio Cassette Tapes

__ Tape 1 - "Body Awareness & Pool Exercise".................$15.36
    By Sheila Cluff
__ Tape 2 - "Stomach, Hips and Thighs"...........................$15.36
    By Sheila Cluff
__ Tape 4 - "Splash N' Stretch"...$15.36
    By Elizabeth Horton
__ Tape 5 - "Stretching and Body Awareness" & "Yoga"...$15.36
    By Eleanor Brown
__ "Sheila Cluff's Aerobic Walking Workout"....................$13.12
    By Sheila Cluff
__ "Abs, Buns & Backs and Water Works"..........................$15.36
    By Elizabeth Horton
__ "Restorative Yoga & Stretching For All Fitness Levels"$15.36
    By Sally Wolpe and Maura Patrice
__ "Chair Yoga and Body Awarness".................................$15.36
    By Sheila Cluff and Eleanor Brown

Video Tapes

__ "Body Awareness With Sheila"......................................$34.90
__ " Low Impact Workout" with Marilu Rogers.................$34.90

Vitamins

__ Multiple Vitamin & Mineral Program(60 day supply)...$31.95

PLEASE TURN THIS PAGE OVER FOR ORDERING INFORMATION

Please send the following information at no charge:

__ The Oaks at Ojai & The Palms at Palm Springs Brochures
__ Travel and Cruise Information
__ Newletter and Calendar of Specials and Events for The Oaks and The Palms

Payments Method (NO CASH PLEASE):

___ Check (Please use an envelope)
___ Visa ___ Mastercard ___ Discover

Card Number:_____Exp. Date:_____

Signature_____

Name (Please Print):_____

Address:_____

City:_____ State:_____ Zip:_____

Phone: (   )_____-_____

All prices include tax, postage and handling
(allow 2-3 weeks for delivery).

Fit Two Inc.
122 East Ojai Avenue
Ojai, California 93023
Attention: Order Desk
Phone: (805) 646-5573 ext. 154
Fax: (805) 646-9392
Web Site: http://www.keho.com/oaks

PLEASE SEE REVERSE SIDE OF THIS PAGE FOR MORE PRODUCTS